Arrhythmias in Children

Arrhythmias in Children
A Case-Based Approach

Vincent C. Thomas

*Pediatric Cardiologist and
Electrophysiologist Medical Safety Officer
Johnson & Johnson
Irvine, CA, United States*

Seshadri Balaji

*Professor
Department of Pediatrics, Division of Cardiology
Oregon Health and Science University
Portland, OR, United States*

ELSEVIER

Elsevier
Radarweg 29, PO Box 211, 1000 AE Amsterdam, Netherlands
The Boulevard, Langford Lane, Kidlington, Oxford OX5 1GB, United Kingdom
50 Hampshire Street, 5th Floor, Cambridge, MA 02139, United States

Notices

Knowledge and best practice in this field are constantly changing. As new research and experience broaden our understanding, changes in research methods, professional practices, or medical treatment may become necessary.

Practitioners and researchers must always rely on their own experience and knowledge in evaluating and using any information, methods, compounds, or experiments described herein. In using such information or methods they should be mindful of their own safety and the safety of others, including parties for whom they have a professional responsibility.

To the fullest extent of the law, neither the Publisher nor the authors, contributors, or editors, assume any liability for any injury and/or damage to persons or property as a matter of products liability, negligence or otherwise, or from any use or operation of any methods, products, instructions, or ideas contained in the material herein.

Library of Congress Cataloging-in-Publication Data
A catalog record for this book is available from the Library of Congress

British Library Cataloguing-in-Publication Data
A catalogue record for this book is available from the British Library

ISBN: 978-0-323-77907-4

For information on all Elsevier publications visit our website at
https://www.elsevier.com/books-and-journals

Publisher: Dolores Meloni
Acquisitions Editor: Robin R. Carter
Editorial Project Manager: Megan Ashdown
Production Project Manager: Niranjan Bhaskaran
Cover Designer: Alan Studholme

Typeset by TNQ Technologies

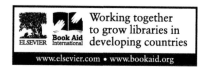

Preface

Managing a pediatric patient with an arrhythmia can be intimidating. It may be the rapid heartbeat, the cardiac involvement, or the potentially serious outcome that creates a sense of unease in the healthcare provider. *Arrhythmias in Children: A Case Based Approach* was written to address these concerns and to provide a simple and logical method to manage the pediatric patient with challenging arrhythmias. The audience for this book is intended for the first-line provider who would encounter these patients including pediatricians, family medicine physicians, emergency room physicians, nurse practitioners, nurses, residents, and medical students. While those training or trained in pediatric cardiology may also find benefit from reading this text, this book does not provide the accustomed detailed and extensive review that other pediatric electrophysiology texts offer.

The primary purpose of this book is to provide a glimpse into the mind of the pediatric electrophysiologist when encountering common clinical scenarios. Each chapter starts with a clinical case that represents our most common clinical experiences in which a healthcare provider is consulting a pediatric electrophysiologist. The reader will find immediately following the clinical case presentation a chapter segment entitled *What am I Thinking?* The segment is purposefully written in a type of "stream of consciousness" using colloquial and emotive language to provide a sense of how a subject matter expert views the situation. It was written to provide the reader with insight into the unfiltered and initial impressions of a pediatric electrophysiologist to provoke thoughts about the next steps, what to look for, and when to be worried.

The book is sectioned into *Infant, Child, and Adolescent* to illustrate arrhythmias and arrhythmia syndromes commonly encountered by age. The final book section is *Special Circumstances* where arrhythmia cases are specific to disease states and less commonly encountered by the general provider. The reader will note that the first three book sections have a similar structure to the chapters with the last book section focusing on case specifics. In the first three sections of the book, the *What am I Thinking* segment is often followed by a differential diagnosis table arranged by likelihood based on the clinical presentation from the viewpoint of the electrophysiologist. Differential diagnoses can be vast and while they should be all inclusive, context to the clinical scenario is key. For those chapters where the diagnosis is known, the differential diagnosis table is replaced with a table germane to the topic. This is followed by chapter segments of *History & Physical, Diagnostic Tests,* and *Action Plan*. The reader will note that in various chapters the discussion will tangent from the clinical case to a general electrophysiology topic for further examination. Readers may find in-depth discussion on pediatric electrocardiogram interpretation (Chapter 8), cardiac ablation (Chapter 9), adolescent syncope (Chapters 16—18), or controversies over screening electrocardiograms (Chapter 11) helpful in their learning. In the final book section of *Special Circumstances*, the chapter ends with a longer version of *What am I Thinking* where specifics of the case are discussed as the questions posed are direct and the underlying diagnosis is known.

It is our sincere hope that this book helps demystify arrhythmias in children by providing key insights into patient management. Learning when and when not to be concerned is the first step of all arrhythmia management in pediatrics. We hope that the lessons learned from this book will add to your efforts to provide quality, safe, and compassionate care for our patients.

Acknowledgments

Vincent C. Thomas
My sincere thanks:

To my wife and children for their unconditional love and support.
To my parents for instilling values of faith and hard work.
To my brothers and extended family for their words of encouragement.
To my mentors and colleagues for their guidance and sage advice.

And to my patients and their families for allowing me to be a part of their lives and for the lessons they have bestowed.

Seshadri Balaji
Dedicated to my parents Parvathavardhini Seshadri and Venkatraman Seshadri.

Contents

Infant

Newborn nursery infant that has bradycardia

Case

I'm calling from the newborn nursery and I'm the charge nurse on for today. I have a 1-day old newborn infant that on auscultation has a slow heart rate. I counted an average pulse rate of 90 beats per minute. The baby looks well and seems to be feeding OK. I've called the pediatrician and she's coming to see the baby this afternoon after clinic, but she asked me to call you. Anything I should be worried about?

What am I thinking?

As with any arrhythmia, the first thing I think about is the clinical status of the patient. In this situation, is the bradycardia impacting the ability of this newborn to live—namely maintaining homeostatic metabolism, eating, and gaining weight? A patient who is not acidotic, able to feed, and is gaining an appropriate amount of weight is less of a concern for immediate intervention. Once I have established that the patient is clinically OK, I need to understand the rhythm and I will be looking for some form of tracing, best performed with a 15-lead ECG. The most common reason an electrophysiologist gets involved for bradycardia in a newborn is sinus bradycardia, which often is a sign of other issues rather than the diagnosis. As long as the patient is clinically stable, I have time to perform a work-up.

Arrhythmias in Children. https://doi.org/10.1016/B978-0-323-77907-4.00001-9

Differential diagnosis

Likely

Sinus bradycardia
- Secondary to respiratory pauses or apnea
- Secondary to maternally administered medications

Possible

Blocked premature atrial contractions
Sinus bradycardia secondary to induced hypothermia

Rare

Congenital hypothyroidism (sinus bradycardia)
Congenital heart block
Long QT syndrome (sinus bradycardia, 2:1 atrioventricular block)
Sick sinus syndrome or heterotaxy syndrome (left atrial isomerism) secondary to congenital heart disease

---

History and physical

History is paramount in the work-up of a newborn infant with bradycardia. While this may seem counterintuitive given the short history outside of the womb, the history should involve what occurred antenatally and in the immediate postnatal period. Foremost, what is the clinical status of the patient? This should always be the first concern in any arrhythmia case and should drive decision-making and actions. Any suggestion of instability due to bradycardia may require immediate action with the consultation of a pediatric cardiologist and preferably, a pediatric electrophysiologist. With a clinically stable patient, history questions may help with diagnostic considerations. Most cases of neonatal bradycardia are due to sinus bradycardia (see Fig. 1.1). Causes of sinus bradycardia can include respiratory-related issues such as apnea of prematurity and/or respiratory pauses. Sinus bradycardia could also be the result of medication given during or after delivery. Bradycardia during fetal life may suggest blood flow insufficiency from the placenta or underlying genetic predisposition such as congenital heart disease or Long QT syndrome. It may also suggest an underlying arrhythmia such as blocked atrial premature beats (see Figs. 1.2 and 1.3). The most common ectopic arrhythmia noted in the normal newborn is that of atrial premature beats. In the neonate with congenital heart block, there is a higher incidence of maternal lupus and this history should be elicited.

On physical examination, most neonates with stable bradycardia have no other significant changes to vital signs. Pauses in respiration leading to bradycardia should be monitored and documented. Any evidence for cyanosis or low oxygen saturation may suggest underlying congenital heart disease. Overall appearance should indicate adequate perfusion and no evidence for skin mottling in a clinically stable neonate. Cardiac murmurs in addition to an expected bradycardic rate may indicate possible congenital heart disease. Irregularity to the rhythm on auscultation may indicate blocked atrial premature beats.

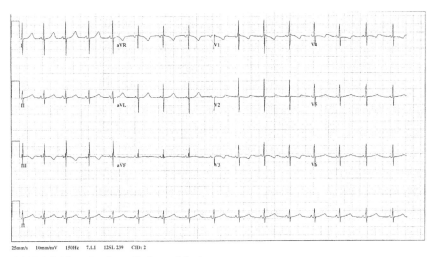

25mm/s   10mm/mV   150Hz   7.1.1   12SL 239   CID: 2

FIGURE 1.1 Sinus bradycardia in an infant.

The ECG demonstrates a bradycardic rhythm around 95 bpm in a newborn infant. There are clear p waves with 1:1 conduction and an appropriate vector for sinus bradycardia. This sinus bradycardia was due to maternal medications given before delivery.

Diagnostic testing

The primary test for bradycardia in the newborn is the electrocardiogram and should be the first test ordered. If bradycardia appears intermittently, the neonate should be placed on a form of continuous monitoring, preferably one with an ability to record the change in rhythm and can capture a single or multi-lead rhythm strip. If such a

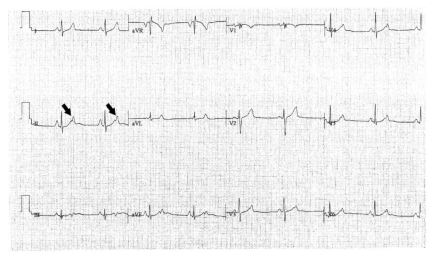

FIGURE 1.2 Blocked premature atrial contractions.

The ECG demonstrates premature atrial beats (arrows) that lie within the T wave and are not conducted to the ventricle resulting in a reduced heart rate.

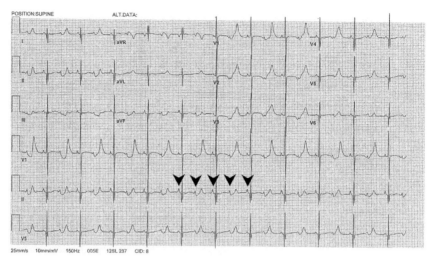

FIGURE 1.3 Long QT syndrome with 2:1 AV block in a newborn.

The ECG demonstrates sinus rhythm with a severely prolonged QT interval that leads to 2:1 conduction of the sinus rate (arrowheads) and subsequent bradycardic ventricular rhythm. Findings of 2:1 conduction due to long QT syndrome in the newborn are very concerning and carry a poor prognosis.

system does not exist in the hospital setting, a Holter monitor may act as a surrogate though requires time for interpretation and action would be delayed by at least 24 h. If there are clinical concerns for congenital heart disease, an echocardiogram should be performed to evaluate the cardiac anatomy. For concerns of congenital heart block, maternal lupus antibodies (anti-SSA, anti-SSB) can be measured. Congenital hypothyroidism is routinely checked in the newborn screen within the United States and should be assessed if there are concerns.

Action plan

As stated previously, the clinical status of the patient is paramount to all arrhythmia management. In a scenario where the patient is clinically not doing well, immediate intervention is often required. Immediate consultation with cardiology is highly recommended. Suggested treatments may include the use of chronotropic medications (e.g., epinephrine, isoproterenol, atropine) or temporary pacing. Temporary pacing can be conducted with the transvenous placement of a temporary pacing lead in the right ventricle and connection with a temporary pacemaker. In emergent situations, temporary pacing can be conducted via defibrillator patch placement on standard hospital cardioverter defibrillators and should always be used with appropriate sedation as external pacing can be quite painful.

A few notes about external cardiac pacing. First, always ensure that the pacing stimuli are indeed creating a conducted beat and not just the appearance of one on the cardiac monitor. Assessment of the *perfusing* rate can be measured in a variety of ways including auscultation, feeling for a central pulse, or use of a pulse oximeter for calculation of the rate. Second, take the opportunity to learn about your hospital cardioverter-defibrillator and how to set the appropriate settings. This piece of life-saving hospital equipment is often used in true emergencies where time is of the essence and should not be first introduced during a patient experiencing a life-threatening arrhythmia. Please note, an automated external defibrillator as seen in the community *does not* have a setting for external pacing.

Most commonly, the patient presenting with bradycardia in the newborn period is demonstrating sinus bradycardia and is clinically stable. The bradycardia is usually a sign of sedation, maternal medications, or possibly respiratory issues. While the first two are self-limited and usually resolve with time, respiratory concerns may best be addressed with supplemental oxygen or air, particularly in the premature infant. Sinus bradycardia is nearly always seen in premature infants who have undergone induced hypothermia for neurologic protection. The ECG often demonstrates a prolonged QT interval and usually resolves once hypothermia is reversed.

In some instances, bradycardia may be due to blocked premature atrial beats in which the atrial beat is not conducted to the ventricle resulting in a lower perfusion rate. Premature atrial beats are one of the more common arrhythmias seen in the newborn and are often benign without clinical impact. Signs that premature atrial beats are benign include single p wave morphology, no evidence for sustained atrial tachycardia, and structurally normal heart. Most often these are seen in patients with structurally normal hearts though an echocardiogram may be helpful to rule out congenital heart disease. In rare instances, what may appear as a premature atrial beat may reflect a single reentrant beat of supraventricular tachycardia. These types of "echo beats" eventually manifest as short runs of supraventricular tachycardia with continued monitoring. Management of newborns with benign premature atrial beats does not require medical treatment and usually monitored with most self-resolving by 6 months of age.

In rare instances, newborns may have more insidious presentations of complex disease manifesting as bradycardia and consultation with a pediatric cardiologist is recommended. Congenital hypothyroidism may present as sinus bradycardia and appropriate treatment should resolve the rhythm. Congenital heart disease, particularly entities with left atrial isomerism may present with a low atrial or junctional escape rhythm due to the lack of a true sinus node (see Fig. 1.4). Most often left atrial isomerism is accompanied with other structural heart defects and often presents with cyanotic heart disease. Newborns with long QT syndrome may present with bradycardia in fetal life. This may be secondary to sinus bradycardia or a 2:1 AV conduction block. Family history of sudden cardiac arrest should be thoroughly evaluated and diagnosis is often established with genetic testing.

Newborns with congenital heart block are often discovered in fetal life due to bradycardia (see Fig. 1.5). Management usually involves a team of an obstetrician, perinatologist, neonatologist, fetal cardiologist, and pediatric electrophysiologist. In rare instances, a newborn may be discovered to have congenital heart block postpartum and management depends on the clinical stability of the patient. Usually,

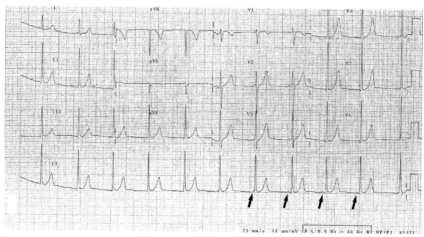

FIGURE 1.4 Junctional rhythm.

The ECG demonstrates an accelerated junctional rhythm just over the rate of the sinus node. Toward the end of the rhythm strip, there are sinus P waves (*arrows*) accelerating over the junctional rate thereby taking over as the dominant rhythm.

careful observation is the first step with a determination of the need for pacemaker based on symptoms, average heart rate, long pauses in cardiac rhythm, and the presence of congenital heart disease. Early consultation with a pediatric electrophysiologist is highly recommended.

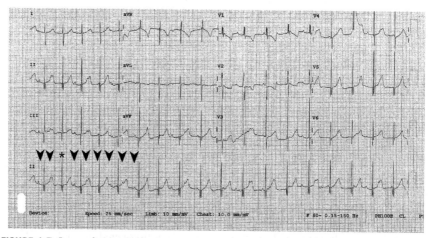

FIGURE 1.5 Congenital heart block.

The ECG demonstrates congenital heart block with a junctional escape rate of approximately 110 bpm. The sinus rate is determined by the rate of P waves (arrowheads) marching through the junctional rate at approximately 165 bpm. The P wave may be buried within the QRS (asterisk).

NICU infant noted to have extrasystoles on cardiac monitor

2

Case

You receive a call from the neonatal intensive care unit (NICU) regarding an ex-34 week premature infant. "I have this 1 week old male infant who is here for a persistent oxygen requirement and feeding issues. The baby was intubated after delivery but now has weaned to 1 liter of oxygen via nasal cannula. The baby has been on parenteral nutrition but is receiving some feeds via nasogastric tube. Because he is on oxygen, he requires monitoring and we have noted extra beats that causes his monitor to alarm. Could you come by and take a look?"

What am I thinking?

Alarms can be the bane of the NICU nurse's existence. Bedside monitors can alarm for a number of reasons, both medical and nonmedical. Usually, extrabeats on the monitor indicate some form of rhythm change in a newborn, but not always. Sometimes, it is related to an artifact that is picked up as an extrabeat. Most often, I usually think the extra beat is a reflection of a premature beat such as a premature atrial beat that is conducted and causes a change in rhythm. Next, I begin to think about the potential etiologies of that atrial premature beat. Does this baby have a low potassium? Does the baby have an umbilical venous catheter or central line that has moved into the right atrium? Lastly, I consider management that often is noncardiac in nature.

Arrhythmias in Children. https://doi.org/10.1016/B978-0-323-77907-4.00002-0

Differential diagnosis
Likely
Atrial premature beat
Artifact
Possible
Ventricular premature beat
Rare
Congenital heart disease
Cardiac tumor

History and physical

Infants in the NICU, by definition, require intensive care that may lead to a clinical setup for monitoring combined with idiopathic changes. Extrabeats noted on the monitor and causing alarms should be reviewed as to the frequency of these occurrences. Additionally, it is important to identify specific time frames where the extra beats are noted (e.g., after medication or after feedings). Given the possible etiologies for premature beats, further history into potential electrolyte disturbances or presence of a newly placed central line should be obtained.

Physical exam should focus on auscultation of changes in rhythm associated with the extra beats noted on the monitor. On some occasions, the change in monitor is not reflected by a change in auscultation but more accurately reflects an artifact due to movement such as with hiccoughs. Auscultation should also focus on the presence of murmurs for congenital heart disease or the exceedingly rare "tumor plop" sound of an atrial myxoma. The presence of any central venous catheters should also be noted.

Diagnostic tests

The first step in the investigation is a review of the monitor. As mentioned earlier, the artifact may lead to the alarm based on the monitor's interpretation of patient movement as a cardiac signal. A useful tip to determine if the signal is cardiac in origin or artifact is to determine the impact on the underlying rhythm. For true cardiac signals, the underlying rhythm is most often impacted resulting in a change in cadence. For artifact, the cadence or rate of the rhythm from beat to beat is unchanged. On occasion, the artifact can be seen transposed on top of a true cardiac signal without any change in underlying rhythm (see Fig. 2.1).

If the monitor is indeed picking up a premature or extra beat, an electrocardiogram is the most useful test given that the rhythm change occurs with enough

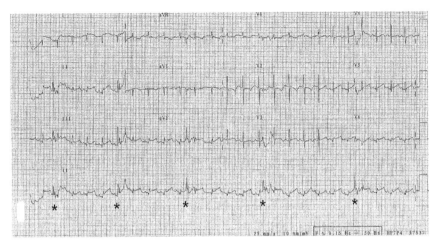

FIGURE 2.1　Artifact from hiccoughs.

The ECG demonstrates sinus rhythm in an infant with a noted artifact (asterisks) that mimics an ectopic beat. The significant clue that the waveforms are artifacts is that there is no change to the underlying rhythm and careful examination demonstrates the normal waveforms marching through the tracing.

frequency to be caught. For atrial premature beats, there are a number of etiologies that may lead to this finding. In the premature infant, electrolyte disturbances are common, particularly those who are on diuretics or require parenteral nutrition. Low serum potassium, magnesium, and calcium can commonly result in atrial premature beats and sometimes ventricular premature beats. For patients with central venous lines, a line that lies deep in the atrium may induce atrial premature beats. This can usually be determined by chest radiograph. For NICU patients with atrial premature or ventricular premature beats, an echocardiogram may be indicated to evaluate for congenital heart disease.

Action plan

Clearly, in the scenario of motion artifact, there are no actions required. When encountering true premature beats in this population, actions are driven by the underlying etiology. Electrolytes should be corrected if there are any abnormal findings on the chemistry panel to see if the extrasystoles resolve. For those neonates with central venous lines that appear deep, the line should be repositioned, replaced, or removed. Congenital heart disease should be managed with the consultation of a pediatric cardiologist.

For those neonates with a structurally normal heart and atrial premature beats without specified etiology, management is heavily based on observation. Isolated atrial premature beats are of little concern and resolve over time (usually by 6 months

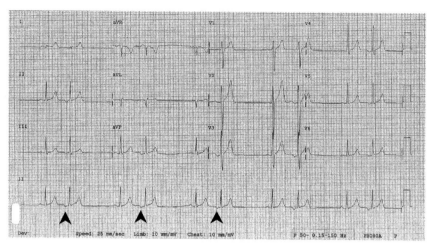

FIGURE 2.2 Premature atrial beats, conducted.

The ECG demonstrates premature atrial beats (arrowheads) that are conducted. They occur every other beat and are therefore the rhythm is termed "atrial bigeminy."

of age) and antiarrhythmic medications are reserved for forms of atrial tachycardia (see Fig. 2.2). NICU neonates with possible atrial tachycardia are often discoverable with monitoring.

Neonates presenting with ventricular premature beats are less common than atrial premature beats. Similarly, these patients deserve monitoring and should be evaluated for any signs of ventricular tachycardia. Increased burdens of premature ventricular beats may lead to ventricular dysfunction. Therefore, baseline echocardiography should be obtained and followed if the burden of premature ventricular beats is relatively high. Medications are usually avoided and reserved for patients with hemodynamic impact or cardiac dysfunction secondary to the ventricular premature beat. This is a rare scenario but should be suspected if the child is in a bigeminal rhythm with the premature beat producing a low stroke volume such that there is effectively a severe bradycardia at half the noted heart rate (see Fig. 2.3). Most neonates will have ventricular premature beats that will self-resolve with time. Consultation and follow-up with a pediatric cardiologist or electrophysiologist are recommended for this group.

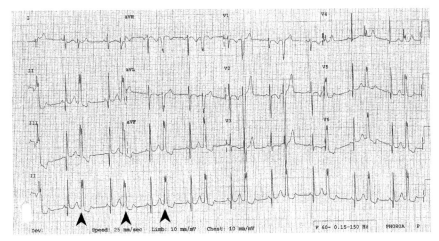

FIGURE 2.3 Premature ventricular beats.

The ECG demonstrates premature ventricular beats (arrowheads). As they occur every other beat, the rhythm is termed "ventricular bigeminy." The morphology of the premature beat is positive in the inferior leads suggesting a ventricular outflow tract origin.

Full-term infant noted to have persistent tachycardia

3

Case

Hi, I'm calling to let you know about a newborn infant that is full-term but transferred to the NICU because of a persistent tachycardia that was noted after delivery. The heart rate seems to remain high regardless of what the baby is doing. The baby seems stable to me, but the heart rate is definitely higher than I would expect. We have an ECG of it but, I have to admit, it's a bit hard for me to interpret.

What am I thinking?

Usually, when I get a call like this, I am thinking about a few different types of tachycardia. A few of the key points in this call are as follows: (1) the baby is stable, (2) the baby is a full-term newborn, (3) the tachycardia has persisted since delivery. Perhaps a bit more subtle are the comments made by the caller that often strikes me as telling. Stating that a heart rate is "higher than I would expect" usually clues me in to consider heart rates that could be considered within the normal range. Often, when a patient has a more typical accessory pathway-mediated, reentrant, supraventricular tachycardia, the heart rate is what the caller leads with (i.e., heart rate is 220 bpm). Here, I am receiving the clue that the heart rate is not that high. Another comment is that the ECG is a "bit hard for me to interpret" suggesting that the ECG does not look entirely normal but it is not obvious that it is abnormal. These types of cases can be exciting for an electrophysiologist (EP) as we rely heavily on our diagnostic capabilities, utilizing our knowledge of arrhythmias, diagnostic maneuvers, and ECG tracings.

Differential diagnosis

Likely

Atrial flutter
Atrioventricular reentrant tachycardia, accessory pathway-mediated
Sinus tachycardia secondary to sepsis or hypovolemia

Possible

Automatic atrial ectopic tachycardia
Multifocal atrial tachycardia
Congenital junctional ectopic tachycardia
Atrioventricular nodal reentrant tachycardia
Persistent junctional reciprocating tachycardia

Rare

Ventricular tachycardia
Sinus tachycardia secondary to hyperthyroidism

History and physical

As with any newborn tachycardia, it is important to establish the onset of the tachycardia. Was the tachycardia noted in fetal life? Immediately after delivery? Sudden onset later in the newborn period? Fetal tachycardias often reflect atrial arrhythmias but can also represent pathway mediated tachycardias and others. On many occasions, the fetal atrial arrhythmia resolves and does not recur after delivery—but this is not always the case. If the arrhythmia was noted only immediately after delivery, the possibility of atrial flutter should be strongly considered. In general, arrhythmias that have a sudden onset later in the newborn period are more suggestive of a reentrant form of tachycardia. History should also elicit any history of maternal infection or fever to evaluate for potential sepsis. Feeding history and assessment of urine output can be helpful to determine volume status and a compromise of the cardiac output.

Characteristics of the arrhythmia itself can assist in determining its etiology. At this time, it would be prudent to review some basic concepts of arrhythmias to further assist in the understanding, diagnosis, and management of pediatric arrhythmias.

Pediatric arrhythmias can be categorized by the arrhythmia mechanism: namely reentrant, automatic, or triggered. The most common mechanism in the pediatric patient is reentry (>90%), followed by automatic (~10%) and triggered as a distant third. Reentrant arrhythmias can be reflected by the circuitous nature of the propagation of the arrhythmia, usually around an anatomic or electrophysiologic barrier (see Fig. 3.1). Given a specified path of the reentrant arrhythmia, there is often minimal to no variation in arrhythmia rate and is reflected clinically as a persistent

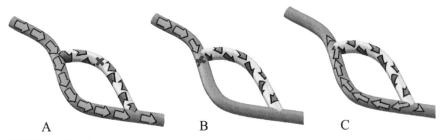

A   B   C

FIGURE 3.1 Reentry.

Reentrant rhythms require two pathways around a functional barrier with differing conduction and recovery properties and unidirectional block. In the figures, the blue pathway represents a "fast" conducting pathway with slower recovery. The yellow pathway represents a "slow" conducting pathway with faster recovery. (A) *Sinus rhythm-* During a sinus beat, the electrical waveform is propagated antegrade along the fast pathway (direct *green arrows*) and slow pathway (spiraling *orange arrows*) simultaneously. Due to the fast conduction of the blue pathway, the waveform reaches the distal end of the yellow pathway and begins to propagate retrograde. The antegrade and retrograde waveforms collide (red X) thereby terminating and preventing reentry. (B) *Premature beat-* A premature beat propagates antegrade and finds the fast pathway refractory due to its slower recovery and is unidirectionally blocked antegrade (red X). However, the waveform finds the slow pathway recovered and propagates slowly (spiraling orange arrows). (C) *Reentrant beat-* When the waveform reaches the distal end of the slow pathway (yellow), it finds the fast pathway capable of conducting retrograde thereby completing the reentrant circuit. This form of slow-fast reentry results in nearly simultaneous activation of the distal and proximal ends connected to the pathway (green arrowheads) as would be seen in AV nodal reentry tachycardia with atrial and ventricular activation.

rate with sudden start and stop. Automatic tachycardias, in contrast, originate as the insidious firing of a group of myocardial cells. As there is no specified path for the arrhythmia to propagate, the rate can vary and often can be subject to the influence of the catecholamine state. This typically presents clinically as a "warm up" or "cool down" variation in heart rate that can be exacerbated by physiologic stress and alleviated with a resolution of physiologic stress (i.e., sedation).

The most common presentation of an atrial flutter in the newborn is a tachycardia that persists and does not change in rate (see Fig. 3.2). In most scenarios, the rate of the atrial flutter tachycardia is twice or three times the ventricular rate due to blocking of the atrial arrhythmia by the atrioventricular node. Sudden onset is more suggestive of a reentrant form of arrhythmia whereas a "warm up" or "cool down" is more suggestive of an automatic ectopic tachycardia, including that of sinus tachycardia.

For the typical newborn presenting with arrhythmia, the physical examination is generally unremarkable. Physical examination should focus for signs of congenital heart disease such as cyanosis, murmur, hepatomegaly, or diminished femoral

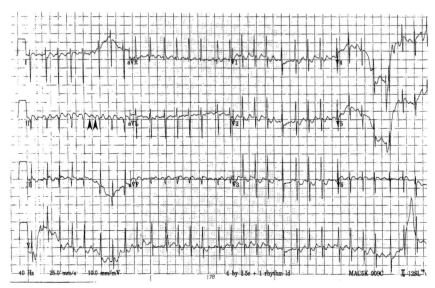

FIGURE 3.2 Newborn atrial flutter.

The ECG demonstrates atrial flutter in a newborn patient. The characteristic "saw-tooth" pattern of the P waves is noted but can be difficult to visualize when masked by the QRS. Spontaneous block of AV conduction may reveal two consecutive P waves providing a diagnosis (arrowheads).

pulses. Other critical signs to evaluate on exam would be for hypovolemia including sunken anterior fontanelle, sunken eyes, poor skin turgor, diminished pulses overall, and prolonged capillary refill. For potential sepsis concerns, the clinician should be assessing overall clinical status including evaluation for signs of infection such as fever, flushed appearance, or rapid capillary refill suggestive of "warm shock," diminished pulses overall, and petechiae/purpura.

Diagnostic testing

The most critical test to order in assessing arrhythmias is the electrocardiogram. While the electrocardiogram can be difficult to interpret at times, a tracing of the rhythm can provide the diagnosis or provide clues to appropriately identify the arrhythmia.

In the clinical scenario described, the caller describes an electrocardiogram that is challenging to interpret. There are a number of methods to assist in the clinical interpretation of arrhythmias, including changes that can be made on the ECG machine itself when collecting the data or in postprocessing. Typical paper speed for an electrocardiogram is 25 mm/s. For rapid arrhythmias, it can be helpful to alter the paper speed to 50 mm/s such that identification of waveforms or changes in

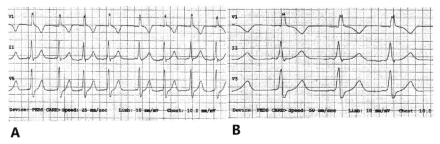

FIGURE 3.3 ECG paper speed.

(A) Electrocardiogram of a patient with Wolff-Parkinson-White taken at 25 mm/s paper speed. This is the standard speed. (B) Electrocardiogram of the same patient running at 50 mm/s paper speed. Note the widening of the waveforms and lengthening of each segment to twice that of standard 25 mm/s paper speed.

rhythm may be easier to interpret (see Fig. 3.3). Standard voltage for the electrocardiogram is 10 mm/mV. It may be difficult to visualize waveforms, particularly atrial tracings. Utilizing a 20 mm/mV setting may allow for better visualization (see Fig. 3.4).

For those patients with noted supraventricular tachycardia, an echocardiogram is reasonable to establish baseline cardiac function and ensure there is no evidence for congenital heart disease. In most cases, the echocardiogram will be normal including the expected finding of a patent foramen ovale in the newborn.

Action plan

Using our understanding of arrhythmia mechanisms combined with our review of the electrocardiogram can help us determine the best course of action.

As mentioned previously, sudden onset and a persistent tachycardia are very suggestive of a reentrant arrhythmia. When dealing with reentrant arrhythmias, it is important to understand what portions of the heart are involved in the circuit. For arrhythmias such as atrial flutter, the arrhythmia circuit propagates around the tricuspid valve. For accessory pathway-mediated tachycardia, the circuit is large (e.g., macroreentrant) and involves the atrium, atrioventricular node, ventricle, and accessory pathway. Contrast this with atrioventricular nodal reentrant tachycardia in which the entire circuit is configured by the slow and fast pathways of the atrioventricular node. Understanding what is involved in the circuit allows for the appropriate course of action to interrupt or "break" the circuit.

Commonly used interventions to break a reentrant circuit focus on the affecting conduction through the atrioventricular node. Vagal maneuvers act to enhance the parasympathetic activity of the vagus nerve innervation to the heart, slowing conduction and hoping to interrupt the arrhythmia circuit. Adenosine is a commonly used medication with rapid onset and rapid clearance that acts on adenosine

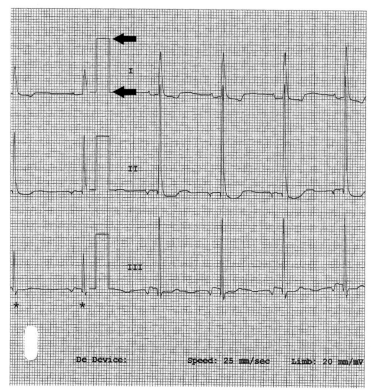

FIGURE 3.4 ECG voltage.

Rhythm strip of leads I, II, and III demonstrates a change in voltage from 10 mm/mV (asterisks) to 20 mm/mV. ECG tracings depict the voltage using a box marker (*arrows*). In this tracing, the box marker is 20 mm or 20 small boxes tall, indicating 20 mm/mV voltage. Note the increase in the size of all the waveforms that allows the user to visualize easier.

receptors primarily at the atrioventricular node, but on other myocardial tissue as well, including the atrium. As these interventions focus on affecting the atrioventricular node, arrhythmia circuits in which the node is involved will be the target of such therapeutic actions (i.e., atrioventricular reentrant tachycardia, atrioventricular nodal reentrant tachycardia) and result in termination of the arrhythmia. It is important to note that although the arrhythmia may terminate, recurrence is still a possibility. Recurrence of reentrant tachycardia may require more long-term management with the use of antiarrhythmic medications such as digoxin or beta-blockers to modify conduction. Consultation with a pediatric electrophysiologist is recommended.

As mentioned in the clinical scenario presented, the electrocardiogram of atrial flutter may be difficult to interpret given the 2:1 conduction and buried P waves within the QRS. Although the atrioventricular node is most certainly not involved in the arrhythmia circuit, further blocking of the conduction from the atrial arrhythmia to the ventricle may allow for clearer identification of the "sawtooth" appearance of atrial flutter (see Fig. 3.5). While adenosine does not interrupt the arrhythmia circuit, it can serve to aid in diagnosis. The same effect can be driven by vagal maneuvers though the resulting AV block is short and less pronounced. Further management for newborn atrial flutter requires cardioversion and should be completed in consultation with a pediatric electrophysiologist. There are a few ways to convert a newborn atrial flutter and this usually involves either the use of esophageal pacing to overdrive pace the flutter or a synchronized cardioversion at 0.5−1 J/kg using the hospital cardioverter-defibrillator. In most cases of newborn atrial flutter, termination of the arrhythmia is straight-forward and recurrence is extremely rare.

Automatic tachycardias are quite challenging to manage. Automatic forms of tachycardia in the newborn include atrial tachycardia, multifocal atrial tachycardia, ventricular tachycardia, and congenital junctional ectopic tachycardia. As there is no circuit to interrupt for these arrhythmias, adenosine or vagal maneuvers have no role. Therapy is focused on suppression with the use of antiarrhythmic drugs and

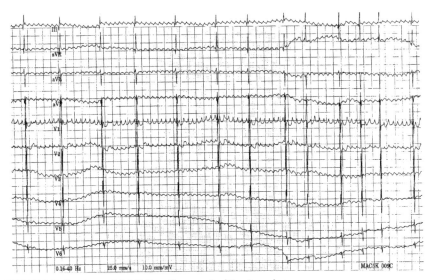

FIGURE 3.5 Newborn atrial flutter diagnosed with adenosine.

Administration of adenosine results in AV block and reveals the atrial flutter pattern more clearly. The ECG demonstrates the same patient from Fig. 3.2 but with a more pronounced AV block due to the administration of adenosine as a diagnostic maneuver. Note that as the AV node is not involved in the reentrant circuit, adenosine does not stop the atrial flutter and is therefore not therapeutic.

2-month-old presenting to the ER with tachycardia, fussy, unable to eat

Case

Hi, I'm calling from the Children's Emergency Room and I have a 6-week-old female that is having tachycardia at a rate of 210 beats per minute (bpm). Baby looks OK but is breathing a little fast and appears a bit mottled. The mother reports that she has not been eating all that well over the past 48 hours and has been fussy. She's only had 3—4 wet diapers over the past 24 hours. There have been some sick contacts at home but not unexpected since we're in the winter season. I'm thinking about giving a fluid bolus but wanted to check with you first. Thoughts?

What am I thinking?

I am worried. There are several reasons for a 2-month-old to have a heart rate above 200 bpm, and none of them are benign. More concerning is the fact that she is presenting to the emergency room and the mother has noted a change. When a mother notes a change in the behavior of their baby, it is generally a good rule to listen, take heed, and investigate. A baby that has not been eating well suggests a problem and if she has a reduction in wet diapers, this concerns me about two possible problems: firstly, her hydration status and secondly, her cardiac output. Breathing fast and a mottled appearance are also concerning signs. Am I dealing with an infection, an undiagnosed congenital heart disease, or a primary arrhythmia? This is a baby I need to monitor carefully, diagnose efficiently, and probably admit to the hospital.

Arrhythmias in Children. https://doi.org/10.1016/B978-0-323-77907-4.00004-4

Differential diagnosis

Likely

Sinus tachycardia
- Secondary to dehydration
- Secondary to infection or sepsis

Supraventricular tachycardia (likely atrioventricular reentrant tachycardia, pathway mediated)

Possible

Sinus tachycardia
- Secondary to congenital heart disease (shunting lesion, ductal dependent lesion)

Supraventricular tachycardia (automatic, atrial ectopic tachycardia)
Supraventricular tachycardia (persistent junctional reciprocating tachycardia)

Rare

Ventricular tachycardia
Inborn error of metabolism

History and physical

Key points to gather in the history surrounding the history of present illness include the start of the clinical status change, the time period over which the decline occurred, and associated symptomatology. All of these can help guide immediate steps in management. A sudden change in clinical status is more indicative of an arrhythmia. Symptoms of illness such as fever, nasal congestion, vomiting, watery stools, and sick contacts would be concerning for infection. A gradual decline in feedings with an increase in respiratory rates over several days could point to undiagnosed congenital heart disease, or a relatively slow but incessant arrhythmia (as can happen with ectopic atrial tachycardia or persistent junctional reciprocating tachycardia). Intolerance to feedings, loss in weight, and changes in neurologic status may be suggestive of metabolic disorder.

The physical exam is critical to diagnosis, with attention to the cardiovascular exam. Evaluation for new cardiac murmur and palpation of femoral pulses should be performed in all infants presenting with tachycardia. Infants between newborn through 3 months are particularly at risk for congenital heart disease presentation due to critical changes in normal human physiology occurring in the transition from fetal circulation.

The first transition from fetal circulation is the normal closure of the ductus arteriosus that usually occurs within hours of birth but can persist to close later, particularly in premature infants and those with "ductal dependent" lesions. "Ductal dependent" refers to the requirement of a persistent ductus arteriosus to supply blood to either the pulmonary or systemic circulation. Pulmonary ductal dependent circulation would present with cyanosis as the ductus closes and can be picked up by monitoring of oxygen saturation. Systemic ductal-dependent circulation, the most common condition being a coarctation of the aorta, would present with a discrepancy of blood flow to the upper and lower half of the body. A discrepancy in pulse between the brachial and femoral pulses should clue the examiner to a ductal dependency.

Another expected physiologic change is the normal drop in pulmonary vascular resistance that usually occurs at 6–8 weeks of life. For those infants with moderate-sized ventricular septal defects or persistent patent ductus arteriosus, the drop in pulmonary vascular resistance can lead to more shunting from the systemic to pulmonary circulation. This can present as a new cardiac murmur and increased respiratory rate due to excessive pulmonary blood flow.

Outside of the cardiovascular examination, there are other signs on physical exam to guide the examiner and assess the clinical status of the infant. General appearance and interaction should be assessed. Infants who present as lethargic, disinterest in latching onto a nipple, grunting respiration, or inconsolable with weak cry and lack of tears are signs of extremis. Evaluate the skin for color, temperature, or rashes. Infants with beads of sweat on the forehead noted during feeding is a sign of congenital heart disease. An enlarged liver may be indicative of congestive heart failure or metabolic disease.

Diagnostic testing

Here again, the clinical status of the patient is paramount. If the patient is presenting in extremis, efforts should be focused on immediate diagnosis and emergent management. For any scenario, the establishment of intravenous access is often required. For those infants that suffer from a reentrant supraventricular tachycardia, placement of the IV can lead to a vagal response and termination of the arrhythmia. The diagnosis of the arrhythmia is predicated on an electrocardiogram tracing however this should never delay management. A recorded or printed monitor rhythm strip may suffice during IV placement.

Any concern for congenital heart disease is best evaluated with an echocardiogram. If concerns are raised for ductal dependent lesions, ordering of prostaglandin to be available at bedside may be efficient management while awaiting the results of the echocardiogram. Cardiac function may be depressed in infants who have been in a sustained arrhythmia for greater than 24 h. Function improves and gradually returns to normal with the conversion to sinus rhythm. Chest radiograph may also be helpful to determine cardiac size, pulmonary blood flow, and evaluate for pulmonary infiltrates. Blood gas, lactate, complete blood count, chemistry panel, and blood culture are other diagnostic labs to consider for work-up. For metabolic disease, additional specialty labs may include serum ammonia, serum amino acids, and urine organic acids.

Action plan

The action plan should depend on the clinical status and underlying diagnosis of the patient. For a patient in extremis, support of clinical needs is of utmost importance including circulation, secure airway, and breathing. In the clinical scenario presented, the emergency room provider has asked about administering a fluid bolus that can be helpful to determine if the tachycardia is secondary to hypovolemia (see Fig. 4.1). Caution should be exercised in providing fluid challenges to patients with congenital heart disease as it may exacerbate congestive heart failure. It is generally recommended to bolus a smaller amount (5 mL/kg) and monitor how the patient responds before giving additional fluid.

Patients with ductal dependency require the use of prostaglandin that should be administered as soon as possible through a secure intravenous line. Those who have suspected infection often require intravenous fluids and antibiotics while carefully monitoring for septic shock. Inotropic agents may be necessary to support blood pressure in the tachycardic infants as acceleration of heart rate serves as the mechanism for increasing cardiac output (heart rate x stroke volume = cardiac output).

For those infants diagnosed with supraventricular tachycardia, termination of the arrhythmia is the primary treatment and choice of treatment methodology should be based on patient status and mechanism of arrhythmia. For the patient in extremis, efforts to convert the rhythm should be expedited. Reentrant arrhythmias may require immediate electrical cardioversion via hospital cardioverter-defibrillator. For those patients suspected of an automatic ectopic tachycardia, immediate

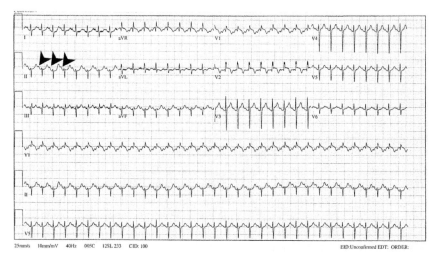

25mm/s   10mm/mV   40Hz   00SC   12SL 233   CID: 100   EID:Unconfirmed EDT: ORDER:

FIGURE 4.1 Sinus Tachycardia.

This ECG demonstrates a long RP tachycardia with the P wave buried in the latter part of the T wave (arrowheads). The P wave has an axis or vector consistent with origination in the sinus node consistent with sinus tachycardia.

consultation with a pediatric electrophysiologist is highly recommended and medication will likely be administered to terminate the arrhythmia while supporting circulation with other measures. This rhythm is due to an abnormal "automatic" focus and will not respond to electrical cardioversion.

If the patient does have some clinical stability, the preferred route for termination of a reentrant arrhythmia would be with the use of adenosine (see Fig. 4.2). As mentioned previously in this text, adenosine works on the adenosine receptors of the myocardial cells, particularly at the atrioventricular node. Adenosine effects are immediate but extremely short as it is immediately metabolized in the bloodstream. Therefore, adenosine should be given through a venous access as centrally located as possible and by fast push that is immediately followed by a generous bolus of saline to make its way through the circulation and back to the heart. The typical dose required is 0.1 mg/kg intravenously up to 6 mg for the first dose. A second dose of 0.2 mg/kg up to 12 mg may be repeated.

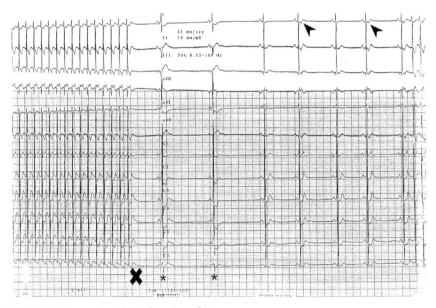

FIGURE 4.2 Diagnosis of SVT with adenosine.

The first part of the ECG demonstrates a narrow complex tachycardiac consistent with SVT, which is terminated (X) with a dose of adenosine. This is followed by two beats (asterisks) of sinus with ventricular preexcitation suggesting an accessory pathway-mediated tachycardia. The following beat demonstrates loss of preexcitation and resumption of conduction down the AV node. The fourth and sixth beat after tachycardia termination demonstrates a retrograde P wave (arrowheads) suggesting reentry through the pathway. The seventh beat again demonstrates reentry immediately preceding the resumption of SVT.

Adenosine always produces an effect. Concerns that the adenosine did not work may reflect that not enough of a dose was given or at a site that was too far away from the heart. Sometimes the anticipated effect of termination of the arrhythmia is not noted because it was short-lived. For this reason, it is highly recommended to perform a rhythm strip electrocardiogram while administering adenosine to monitor and capture the effect. If the clinical status of the patient allows for the administration of adenosine through an intravenous line, there is sufficient time to obtain an electrocardiogram rhythm strip of the event. It is recommended to mark by pen on paper the time the dose was given. Remember that termination of the arrhythmia may be short-lived or may not occur where the atrioventricular node is not a part of the arrhythmia circuit (e.g., ectopic atrial tachycardia, ventricular tachycardia) (see Fig. 4.3). However, diagnostic clues for the electrophysiologist may be available in the rhythm strip that may aid in diagnosis and management.

In patients with a suspected supraventricular arrhythmia, the diagnostic value of the response to adenosine cannot be overstated. Termination of the rhythm abnormality with the resumption of sinus rhythm even if short-lived, is a clue that the AV node is part of the circuit of the tachycardia. In such an event, AV node blocking drugs such as digoxin or β-blockers may help control the rhythm. Alternatively, if adenosine reveals an "atrial" tachycardia such that there are more p waves than

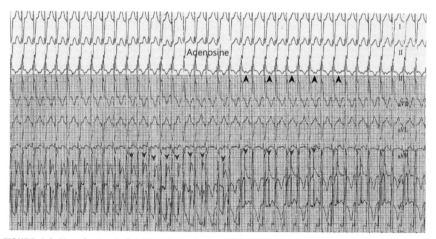

FIGURE 4.3 Ventricular-Atrial (VA) dissociation with adenosine.

Rhythm strip from a postoperative cardiac infant demonstrating a persistent, somewhat narrow complex tachycardia despite the administration of adenosine. Although no change occurs in rhythm, VA dissociation is noted after adenosine administration as seen by dissociated P waves in lead III (black arrowheads). Leads V1 and V2 are attached to atrial pacing wires depicting atrial activity (red arrowheads). A diagnosis of ventricular tachycardia was confirmed with VA dissociation.

QRS complexes while the adenosine is having its effect, that points to a tachycardia arising in the atrium (e.g., ectopic atrial tachycardia or atrial flutter) and the AV node is merely a bystander conveying the rhythm to the ventricle. These non-AV-node-dependent rhythms are harder to control and treat. While flutter can be converted with cardioversion, ectopic atrial tachycardia often does not respond to cardioversion since it is an automatic focus with properties similar to the sinus node, only faster in rate. Imagine cardioverting someone out of sinus tachycardia!

4-month-old with extrasystoles on auscultation at pediatrician's office

---

Case

I have a 4-month old male in my office today for a well-infant check, who is growing well and doesn't appear to have any clinical concerns but when I listen on cardiac exam, I am hearing some extra beats or changes in rhythm that seem a bit off. I'm thinking I should send him to you for evaluation. Should I order an event monitor or something first?

What am I thinking?

The first piece to the presentation is that the baby does not appear to have any clinical concerns which is usually a good sign. Hearing extra beats most commonly presents as a benign finding of a premature atrial beats or possibly premature ventricular beats. Sometimes the extra beat may not have anything to do with a change in rhythm and could represent just an extra auditory sound. Ordering the right test is important, but in an infant this young, obtaining a good family history for any inheritable disease is just as important.

Differential diagnosis
Likely
Premature atrial beats, conducted or blocked
Possible
Premature ventricular beats Single reentrant beat of supraventricular tachycardia, "echo beat"
Rare
Cardiac rhabdomyoma (tuberous sclerosis) Cardiac fibroma Mitral valve click

Arrhythmias in Children. https://doi.org/10.1016/B978-0-323-77907-4.00005-6

History and physical

An infant history can clue any examiner to a potential etiology for extrasystoles noted on examination. Family history is a critical component to any evaluation within pediatrics, but particularly in the world of pediatric cardiology and electrophysiology. Understanding the familial patterns in the pediatric patient allows for a greater understanding for the potential of disease. It is often recommended to conduct a comprehensive family history including a genetic pedigree. As genetic disease may be undiagnosed or not shared with family members, asking questions focused on symptoms may be helpful. For example, obtaining a history for tuberous sclerosis may be focused on not only the existence of the diagnosis itself in the family history but also eliciting a history of seizures. When asking about family history of sudden death, it is helpful to elaborate on different forms including unexplained drownings, unexplained car accidents, or death while playing sports. The art of asking questions is a skill that must be practiced and configured to the clinical scenario. Asking questions surrounding serious conditions that may result in sudden death could raise unnecessary concerns in parents. Therefore, it is advised that asking the right questions should be equally coupled with actively listening for the right answer. Reading the situation, the patient, and the family can mean the difference between being led to a diagnosis versus being led astray.

Auscultation on the cardiac exam is what leads to the noted change in rhythm. Listening for an extended period of time and counting the number of extra beats may be helpful to determine the frequency. Auscultating for other cardiac sounds such as cardiac murmur may help indicate the possible presence of congenital heart disease. Additionally, if the extra beat is heard during every cardiac cycle (systole + diastole), this is likely to indicate a tie to an anatomic etiology. Arrhythmia-related changes usually are accompanied by a pause in rhythm and do not occur with every cardiac cycle. Stigmata for other diseases should be evaluated for physical examination (e.g., Ash Leaf macule).

Diagnostic testing

As mentioned previously, a standard electrocardiogram is the best initial test to order. If there are concerns for the possibility of structural heart disease from history and/or physical examination, an echocardiogram would be diagnostic. In the clinical scenario presented, the physician asks about an event monitor as the appropriate test to order. The answer depends on the frequency of the arrhythmia and the symptomatology presented by the patient. Different types of outpatient monitoring devices can be utilized for the recording of arrhythmias in patients, and a review of these devices is presented.

(1) Holter monitor: A Holter monitor is a continuous monitoring device meaning that the rhythm of the patient will be recorded for the extent that the monitor is

programmed and in contact with the patient. Most Holter monitors present with multiple leads to provide multichannel recording and can record between 24 and 48 h. Most Holter monitors are equipped with a button to signal the presence of a symptom by the patient, however, the button has no impact on the recording. For patients who have frequent rhythm concerns that are short-lived, with or without symptoms, a Holter monitor may be the best choice. Once completed, the monitor is returned for evaluation of all recorded rhythms and a report is provided.

(2) Event monitor: An event monitor is a device that records on a continuous loop and stores the rhythm recorded when a button is pressed indicating when the patient felt a symptom. For those that remain on the skin surface, the total time before pressing the button and after pressing the button can be programmed (e.g., 2 s prerecording, 6 s postrecording) to help provide onset of arrhythmia. Other event monitors that do not remain on the skin surface can be placed on the skin if there are symptoms felt by the patient. These can be helpful in scenarios where the arrhythmia is felt to last for several seconds to minutes allowing time for the patient to obtain the monitor, connect it to the skin, and press the recording button. The onset of arrhythmia would not be recorded in such a scenario; however, the convenience of not wearing the monitor can be a benefit. These monitors are generally administered for 30 days at a time. Some monitors can connect to the monitoring center once a recording is obtained, via either a phone line or internet connection.

(3) Intermediate-term monitoring: In recent years, there have been a number of technological advances that have allowed for the miniaturization of devices coupled with advances in skin adhesion that may allow for longer monitoring times. These devices are inconspicuous but usually accompanied by the trade-off of multi-lead for single-lead recording. Some may connect to a monitoring center while others must be sent after completion of the recording for analysis. Usually, these devices can act as both an event monitor and Holter monitor providing symptom-specific recording along with long-term recording. Monitoring can last anywhere between 2 weeks and 30 days but frequently depends on the length of time that the device is adhered to the skin.

(4) Implantable loop recorder: An implantable loop recorder is a device that is implanted underneath the skin in a surgical procedure that will record under a continuous loop for up to 3 years. Recent advances have allowed the device to reduce in size to that of a large paper clip and only a few millimeters in thickness that can be implanted within minutes. The device can be programmed to monitor for any significant arrhythmias which will record if detected, regardless of patient symptoms. Patients are also provided with an activator that can be placed over the recorder implant location that can activate recording in the case of symptoms. These devices can be interrogated using specified computer systems either in person or from home. While costly, these devices may be helpful in patients who do not have frequent presentations but are potentially at risk for significant or life-threatening arrhythmias.

Action plan

The most common presentation for an infant with extrasystoles is that of premature atrial beats. This is usually diagnosed by electrocardiogram. Premature atrial beats may be conducted or nonconducted (blocked) through the AV node (refer to Chapter 2, Figure 2 and Chapter 1, Figure 2, respectively). Those that are conducted may result in aberrant conduction within the ventricle that may mimic a premature ventricular beat. As previously mentioned, infants with premature atrial beats have a normal prognosis and self-resolve over time. Premature ventricular beats should be monitored but generally also self-resolve. If the beat reflects a single reentrant beat, continued monitoring will often reveal short salvos of supraventricular tachycardia.

Conditions such as cardiac tumors do require regular monitoring and should have the participation of a pediatric cardiologist. In the setting of tuberous sclerosis, these rhabdomyomas will often reduce in size with time and will not require any form of surgical intervention. Rhabdomyomas are mostly located within the ventricle and should be monitored for the development of ventricular arrhythmias. Surgical intervention is reserved for those tubers that interfere with cardiac valve function, hemodynamic consequences, or recalcitrant arrhythmias. Fibromas generally do not reduce in size and often require surgical intervention for removal.

9-month-old with recurrent episodes of supraventricular tachycardia despite medical therapy

Case

Hi, I'm calling about a 9-month old infant, that you follow, with supraventricular tachycardia. She presented today after the parents noted that her heart rate was elevated to our urgent care. Heart rate was steady at about 220 bpm and mom said they first noted it about 2 h ago. We were able to apply ice to the face and forehead a couple of times that seemed to slow it down but really didn't break it. Then as we were getting an IV, the tachycardia broke. Right now, she looks great, comfortable, and has a heart rate of 120 bpm. She is on propranolol and mom says she's been getting her doses. I'd like to send her home but wondering if there is anything you would like me to do?

What am I thinking?

First thing is I am relieved to hear that the tachycardia has broken but now it is a matter of making sure that we prevent it from initiating again. Under these circumstances, I likely have an idea of who this family is and what type of tachycardia I am dealing with. Given the age and heart rate, I am likely dealing with an accessory pathway-mediated reentrant supraventricular tachycardia. It sounds like I have been treating with β-blockers but the one thing about this age is the growth that these infants can experience in a short period of time. I should be thinking about the dose and if it is still appropriate for the infant's size. Given a heart rate of 120 bpm at rest, we may have some room to increase. If not, maybe we try another medication in addition or switch altogether. Ultimately, we have options. Once I have adjusted the medication, it is probably time to bring the family back in and repeat discussions around monitoring and vagal maneuvers.

Arrhythmias in Children. https://doi.org/10.1016/B978-0-323-77907-4.00006-8

Differential diagnosis

Likely

Supraventricular tachycardia
- Accessory pathway mediated, reentrant

Possible

Supraventricular tachycardia
- Atrioventricular nodal reentrant
- Ectopic atrial tachycardia

Rare

Multifocal atrial tachycardia
Ventricular tachycardia
Second form of supraventricular tachycardia
Proarrhythmic effects from medication overdosing

History and physical

Infants who present with recurrence of their tachycardia should start with an evaluation of their current treatment regimen. A single breakthrough episode in a patient with SVT is not a cause for alarm and does not immediately merit a change of plan. For those who are on medication, a clear understanding of the type of medication and the "target" dose when prescribed is essential to understand the next steps. Target dose refers to the dose per body weight or body surface area achieved. As infants undergo rapid growth, this dose is frequently outgrown and thereby interferes with the appropriate steady-state of the medication. A review of any missed dosing or changes in dosing should also be assessed. As the medication provided to infants is a solution or suspension, the concentration of the medication and any pharmacy changes may lead to a change in dosing given that parents often are more cognizant of a medication amount (i.e., milliliters) versus a dose (milligrams). Finally, a review of medication tolerance should be sought with the parents. It is not uncommon for parents to forego medications if they feel that their infant is not tolerating the medication or that there are challenges with administration, including cost.

As with any infant with tachycardia, physical examination should focus on signs of hemodynamic stability to determine the need for immediate action. Temperature, respiratory rate, oxygen saturation, pulses, hepatomegaly, and capillary refill are some of the signs to be evaluated for the possibility of cardiomyopathy secondary to arrhythmia.

Recurrent supraventricular tachycardia (SVT) in an infant can be a source of great anxiety and inconvenience to parents. In general, infants are first diagnosed with SVT after some form of clinical symptomatology that usually involves anxious and hurried visits to medical care. This is usually followed by the initiation of medication and monitoring with equipment not available for home use. Finally, after a return to some level of normalcy for the infant, the parent is quickly educated on the importance of providing these medications on a strict schedule, asked to monitor for any recurrences with limited resources, and to follow up with a heart doctor. Recurrence can be perceived by parents as parenting failure, worsening of condition, or a worsening prognosis—all of which are not true.

Diagnostic testing

The standard electrocardiogram is the best test to assess rhythm and is particularly helpful in the infant with tachycardia recurrence. Presumably, the infant's previous tachycardia has been documented on electrocardiogram and can be utilized for comparison (see Fig. 6.1). Subtle changes in an electrocardiogram may clue the trained electrophysiologist if there are changes in the arrhythmia or if the tachycardia represents a second form. Any attempts to modify or break the tachycardia should be captured on a running rhythm strip, preferably with multiple leads as with a standard electrocardiogram. Documentation of the response of the SVT to vagal maneuvers or drug treatment like adenosine can provide significant clues about the type of arrhythmia and its likely response to therapy.

Echocardiography may be indicated in infants that raise concerns for decreased cardiac function. Additional labs such as a blood gas, electrolyte panel, or drug level (i.e., digoxin level, flecainide level) are dependent on the appearance of the infant and medications elicited in history.

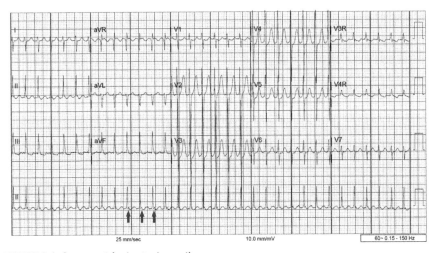

FIGURE 6.1 Supraventricular tachycardia.

The ECG demonstrates narrow complex tachycardia consistent with supraventricular tachycardia. Retrograde P waves (*red arrows*) are noted at the end of the QRS suggesting an accessory pathway-mediated atrioventricular reentrant tachycardia.

Action plan

In the immediate term actions should be driven toward termination and control of the tachycardia. A few words about vagal maneuvers. As indicated in the terminology, vagal maneuvers are those that enact parasympathetic activation of the vagus nerve, leading to a reduction in heart rate and conduction through the atrioventricular node. These maneuvers can be helpful to terminate reentrant forms of tachycardia (see Fig. 6.2).

The most commonly utilized, and often poorly performed, maneuver in the infant or child is the use of ice to the face. The maneuver is intended to induce a "diving reflex." When cold water hits the face, the reflexive action of the vagus nerve to the heart is enacted resulting in bradycardia. To perform this maneuver well, the user must use a resealable plastic bag large enough to cover the entire face containing a mix of ice and water to create a slush. The bag should be rapidly applied (imaging diving into a pool) to the entire face of the patient and for an uncomfortably long period of time, usually 10–15 s. Giving the older child or parent fair warning is highly recommended as the maneuver is visually anxiety provoking and can be mistaken for suffocating. This is not meant to "cool" the patient down as one would perform with a wet cloth to the forehead. An infant will undoubtedly cry vociferously after an ice to the face maneuver, which may also result in a vagal response.

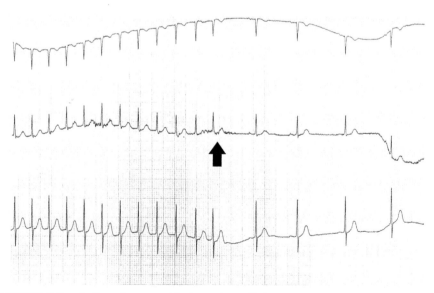

FIGURE 6.2 Termination of supraventricular tachycardia by vagal maneuver.

A rhythm strip demonstrating supraventricular tachycardia that is terminated (*arrow*) by use of a vagal maneuver.

Other maneuvers in infants can include hanging the baby upside down while supporting the head or use of a rectal thermometer for a rectal stimulation. In older children, blowing on the thumb, occluded straw, or syringe while bearing down or Valsalva can be effective. A modification of this maneuver has been proposed by immediately changing position from a seated to a Trendelenburg position, presumably increasing venous return. Doing headstands (with assistance) or somersaults have also been shown to be effective. Drinking an ice-cold beverage while holding one's breath may terminate the arrhythmia as the esophagus lies directly behind the left atrium. Unilateral carotid massage may be helpful in older children as well though a fair amount of pressure should be applied to gain an effect. Older textbooks may advise the use of ocular pressure. This maneuver can cause damage to the eyes and should be avoided. All these maneuvers can be performed in the home setting for the termination of SVT.

In the short term, consultation with the infant's medical team is recommended. All infants with recurrent tachycardia should be assessed and evaluated by a pediatric cardiologist, preferably, electrophysiologist. There may be minor adjustments to medication dosing that can be advised to help prevent recurrences, often accounting for the infant's unaccounted growth. In some instances, medication changes may be warranted, particularly if upper dosing limits have been reached on previous medications. These may require inpatient stays for monitoring as antiarrhythmic drugs may be proarrhythmic. In rare instances, the medication previously used may have led to the presenting arrhythmia due to inappropriate dosing and proarrhythmic effects. In such instances, immediate termination of medication administration, drug levels, electrolyte administration, and binding agents are appropriate next steps.

Once the infant is stabilized, attention is turned to the parents. Recurrent tachycardia is an additional opportunity for parental education. Given the anxiety provoked, it is beneficial to review that infant tachycardia often resolves on its own by 12—15 months old. An opportunity to review medications and how to administer them should be performed. Determine which forms of monitoring are most comfortable for the parents. Home monitoring may range from wearable devices that connect to the parent's smartphone to listening with an ear to the chest after feedings. Finally, emphasize regular follow-up with their pediatrician and the supporting pediatric cardiologist.

Child

2-year-old presents to ER with an episode of "passing out" and "turning blue"

Case

Hi there, sorry to bother you, but I was wondering if I could curbside you on a case I'm seeing in the urgent care? I have a 2-year old who came in with his parents because he passed out at home. He has been otherwise healthy and was running around at home, chasing his older sibling, when he tripped on the rug and hit his head against the coffee table. Parents were in the other room and heard the thud, heard a loud cry. They ran into the room to find him with his mouth agape but no sound, as though he wanted to cry but couldn't make the sound. His face turned blue and then he passed out. He remained blue and out for about a minute or two, according to parents. He then woke up and seems to be OK other than being a little tired according to mom. He has a pretty decent sized abrasion on his forehead so I am sending him to the ER for a CT scan. He's happy and playful again but the passing out and turning blue concerns me. Should I get an echocardiogram or have them meet you in the ER or something?

What am I thinking?

If you have ever seen a child lose consciousness, it can be quite a scene. The vast majority of the time, a syncopal episode in a child can be a benign event but there are a few key findings that can distinguish between a benign situation and a potentially life-threatening one. Hearing a child hitting their head and then finding them on the floor blue is certainly disconcerting for any parent, feels like it lasts forever, and often results in emergent medical follow up. Trying to discern what happened can be difficult when the parent has just gone through a frantic situation. But here is where the astute clinician focuses on gathering all the facts through a very methodical history taking. I often have to redirect parents as they begin to skip over sequences or overestimate the amount of time that passed. Taking a patient and methodical approach to the history of present illness can save a whole lot of worry. Being lucky enough to witness a child breath-holding before passing out nearly cinches the diagnosis.

Arrhythmias in Children. https://doi.org/10.1016/B978-0-323-77907-4.00007-X

Differential diagnosis
Likely
Breath-holding spell
Seizure disorder
Possible
Neurocardiogenic syncope
Munchausen by proxy
Rare
Hypertrophic cardiomyopathy
Catecholaminergic polymorphic ventricular tachycardia
Arrhythmogenic right (or left) ventricular dysplasia
Long QT syndrome
Brugada syndrome

History and physical

A thorough, detailed, and meticulous history is paramount in all cases of syncope, particularly in the young pediatric patient. In many ways, it can be compared to a crime scene investigation in which details are gathered from all eyewitnesses to put together a reenactment of the event in question. These select details can help guide the clinician in the pursuance of further work-up or recognition of a benign condition. Given the importance of such history-taking, it is imperative that the appropriate time be taken (and allotted) for such an evaluation. Part of the evaluation often involves asking questions repeatedly to get a clear answer as patients and parents will often report the main event skipping over multiple details that can help tease out the differential diagnosis.

First, an understanding of the circumstances of the event can be helpful. Was this a typical day or a special event (i.e., sports practice, race day, etc.)? Where was everyone located and who witnessed the event? What was the environmental climate during the event (i.e., hot day outside vs. indoors)? What was the general feeling of the patient before the event: history of previous illness? Appropriate nutrition and hydration that day and days prior? Overall feeling of health? As in the clinical scenario described in the beginning, was there injury, crying, and/or breath-holding that preceded the event? By setting the scene of the environment, we can better understand what may have led up to the event.

Next, turn to the event itself. What was the patient feeling and how were they acting according to eyewitnesses, minutes to seconds before the event? In patients experiencing arrhythmia, it is often reported that the patient was acting unusually before collapse; this is particularly true with sports participants (i.e., shooting an own goal, running the opposite way, standing in an awkward position). How did the patient collapse: were they able to put their hands out to "catch" their fall or did they collapse without doing so leading to injuries? What does the patient recall about the fall: any prodrome of unusual heartbeats, visual changes, or nausea? Many arrhythmia-related syncope patients have no recollection of the event while those who experience a vagal-related syncope often experience symptoms of lightheadedness, dizziness, and/or tunnel-vision without mention of unusual heartbeats. Interestingly, many patients also report nausea, and sometimes describe themselves as feeling hot (sometimes, cold) all over before the event. The total time that the patient was out is often a source of error, as the event often feels longer than by actual time. It may be helpful to ask the observer to walk through the event in their mind while paying attention to the clock. "Reliving" the event can help get a more accurate timing, potentially leading to what was formerly thought of as minutes to seconds. A description that the event lasted longer more than 5 minutes should be a cause for concern. In general, time slows down for concerned parents and a short event that lasted a few seconds can feel like a long time. That said, most parents of patients with benign syncope feel the event was long but not truly over 5 minutes.

After the patient loses consciousness, key questions for eyewitnesses include: was the patient breathing? How did the patient look (i.e., pale, ashen, blue, diaphoretic)? Was there a pulse noted? Was there any shaking of limbs or eye deviation? Was there any urinary incontinence? Were any resuscitative measures used including the use of an automated external defibrillator? If so, were there any tracings from the defibrillator that could be obtained?

Questioning then leads to how the patient regained consciousness and how they felt. Patients who have undergone a significant arrhythmia may not recall much of what happened before passing out and often awaken to discover that something had happened, but they feel ready to return to their previous activity. Those who have suffered a vagal-related syncope often feel fatigued or worn from their bodies having gone through a fight or flight response. Discuss any significant injuries that the patient experienced after their fall. Patients who were able to catch themselves as they fell usually have scratches and bruises on their extremities. Those with arrhythmia who were unable to brace for a fall may result in significant facial injuries such as a broken nose, chipped teeth, and/or hematoma.

Next, history should then transition to the family. Questions should include any family member that suffered an unexplained death such as an unexplained car accident or drowning. Questions should be asked about family members with unexplained seizures or deaths while playing sports—either in practice or in game. Ask about deaths presumed to be due to heart attack before the age of 50 years, which may be in fact a sign of arrhythmic death. Questions should also touch on possible aborted sudden cardiac arrest that usually manifests as syncope in specific situations. For example, asking about family members that pass out with loud noises (long QT syndrome) or with excitement such as roller coasters or being startled/surprised (catecholaminergic polymorphic ventricular tachycardia). Lastly, use medical and colloquial terms to ask about family history. For example, when asking about a family history of hypertrophic cardiomyopathy, also ask if there are any individuals in the family that has been diagnosed with a very thick or enlarged heart. Sometimes descriptions of the disease can trigger memories or commentary from other family members that may be helpful to explore.

Finally, it is advised to take the time to obtain a social history to determine how comfortable the parents and/or patient is at home. Are there any unusual stressors that are affecting the family? Are there any new members living in the household? An opportunity to identify child or spousal abuse should never be missed.

On physical examination of the child, evaluate for any suggestion of cardiac disease in the form of cyanosis at baseline, heart murmur, or abnormal heart rhythm. In the case of breath-holding spells, the physical exam is most often normal. If seizures are high on the differential diagnosis, evaluation of the neurologic status of the child and stigmata of neurologic disorders should be assessed. Signs of abuse should also be evaluated in physical exam. If any evidence for abuse, consult with a child abuse specialist, social services, and/or child protective services to keep the child safe until a more extensive evaluation of the home situation can be performed. While such measures can be time consuming, they can be life saving and, indeed, life altering.

Diagnostic testing

If the history is highly suggestive of breath-holding spell, there are no additional tests to perform. If there are concerns of an arrhythmia syndrome from history, an electrocardiogram is the next most logical test to obtain. This may involve evaluating electrocardiograms on first-degree relatives as well. Any physical examination findings suggestive of anatomic cardiac disease should be evaluated by an echocardiogram. If seizures are a significant possibility, the usual next step is a consultation with a neurologist and likely an electoencephalogram (EEG) with brain imaging (CT or MRI). In cases of suspected abuse, further tests should be in the direction of a child abuse specialist.

Action plan

For the clinical scenario presented, the child presents with a history consistent with a breath-holding spell. Parents should be educated about breath-holding spells being a very anxiety-provoking but generally benign, condition. There is no specific medical treatment for the breath-holding and most patients will outgrow the condition by the age of 5 years. Supportive care is primarily focused on the education of parents and avoiding injury by asking the parents to place the child on the floor as a preemptive measure during a preceding injury that could result in the spell.

If there are concerns regarding a possible cardiac etiology based on thorough history taking and physical examination findings, consultation with a pediatric cardiologist/electrophysiologist is highly recommended. This will often involve an assessment of all first-degree relatives and an extensive family history as conditions are usually genetically inherited.

3-year-old is noted by pediatrician to have a low resting heart rate

Case

Hi, thanks for taking my call. I have a 3 year-old boy in my office today who I am seeing for a well-child check. I have been following him since he was born and he really hasn't had any issues. His parents are great and come in for routine follow ups. He is keeping up with his developmental milestones and he is up to date with all his immunizations. But I am listening to him today and his heart rate seems kind of slow. I don't know what to make of it. His parents say that he is an active three year old and has lots of energy. They have noticed nothing out of the ordinary or concerning to them- but this heart rate just gets me. When I count it out, I get a rate of 70 bpm at rest. We have a blood pressure machine here and he has a normal blood pressure for age, but it reads a heart rate of 65 bpm! What do you think? Should I send him to you for evaluation? Am I missing something?

What am I thinking?

Heart rates in children can be so varied. Here, we have a toddler that is asymptomatic, doing well, growing well, and there is no real concern, but the heart rate was found to be low for age. Here, my advice would be to "trust your gut" because, in most cases, your "gut" is right! The patient's clinical status should always be the guiding principal in any concern for rhythm-related issues and the fact that this toddler is doing well should not alarm us about a low heart rate for age. The lack of symptoms is the key. There are evaluations that we can perform but overall, nothing particularly worrisome here.

Arrhythmias in Children. https://doi.org/10.1016/B978-0-323-77907-4.00008-1

Differential diagnosis
Likely
Sinus bradycardia for age Normal sinus arrhythmia
Possible
Nonconducted premature atrial beats
Rare
2nd or 3rd degree AV block, congenital 2nd or 3rd degree AV block, acquired - Lyme disease - Myocarditis Progressive cardiac conduction disease (Lenégre's disease)

History and physical

As with all potential arrhythmias, the first thing to establish is the symptomatology of the patient. In the scenario of bradycardia, the concern is that the heart rate that drives cardiac output is insufficient. In this rare case, the patient may experience dizziness, fatigue with activity, and/or syncope. Most often, patients are asymptomatic at presentation but any suggestion of inadequate cardiac output warrants further investigation. Eliciting history of a previous viral illness or sick contacts in the prior 2 weeks may suggest a rare myocarditis picture when combined with established conduction disease. Travel history to areas endemic to tick-borne illnesses such as Lyme disease should be obtained. Lastly, the family history of any individuals with conduction disorders with the need for a pacemaker should be asked about.

Physical examination may be entirely normal except for heart rate. Upon auscultation of the heart rate, assessment of the rhythmic beating can be a distinguishing feature. Contrast a consistent sinus bradycardia rate versus that of varying rates related to normal sinus arrhythmia (see Fig. 8.1). Here, the heart rate increases with inspiration and decreases with expiration. A helpful finding is to determine heart rate response to activity. Asking the child to be active and then listening to the heart rate to determine if there is an appropriate tachycardic response is reassuring.

Diagnostic testing

The primary test to order is the electrocardiogram for a diagnostic representation of the heart rhythm. In most pediatric cases, the most common heart rhythm is sinus

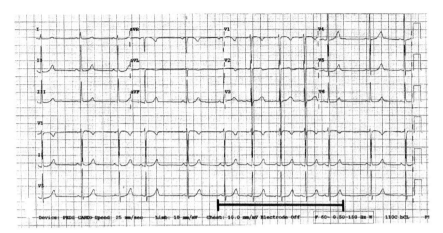

FIGURE 8.1 Normal sinus arrhythmia.

ECG demonstrates normal sinus arrhythmia in which the sinus rate accelerates during inspiration (bracket) and slows during expiration. This reflects a normal physiologic phenomenon and is not an "arrhythmia."

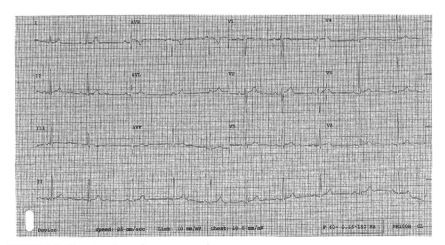

FIGURE 8.2 Sinus bradycardia, normal variant.

ECG demonstrates sinus bradycardia at a rate of approximately 60 bpm. This ECG is taken from an older child but demonstrates the normal P waves consistent with a rhythm originating from the sinus node.

bradycardia (see Fig. 8.2). While this chapter is not intended to be a complete instruction on the interpretation of pediatric electrocardiogram, a basic introduction is provided.

As with most diagnostic tests requiring interpretation, it often helps to have a repeatable pattern, so as not to miss any critical steps. Here, we share a practical approach to electrocardiogram interpretation. However, there is no "single" or "correct" approach but rather, the best method for the interpreter.

First, start with the technical aspects: ensure that the electrocardiogram is for the correct patient and establish the paper speed usually listed at the bottom (25 mm/s is standard); with the appropriate paper speed, each small box is 40 ms and each big box (5 small boxes) is 0.2 seconds with a total time on an electrocardiogram of 6 seconds. Check for voltage either listed on the bottom or depicted as the height of boxes at the end of the strip (10 mm/mV is standard, 20 mm/mV is double, 5 mm/mV is half-standard).

Next, start the interpretation with identification of waveforms and segments. Waveforms should include P waves, QRS complexes, and T waves while segments (also known as intervals) include PR interval, QT interval, and ST segment (see Fig. 8.3). For each waveform, a rate, height (voltage), width (time interval), and vector (axis) is calculated. For each segment, establish the width (time interval) and any elevation or depression from baseline.

Working through the electrocardiogram in this pattern lets cardiac conduction drive the method. Start with the P wave and establish the rate of atrial contractions. Tall P waves suggest right atrial enlargement and wide P waves suggest left atrial enlargement. Ensure that the vector of the P wave is consistent and in line with originating from the sinus node (positive in leads I, II, and aVF). An unusual P wave may indicate that the atrial activation is from a focus other than the sinus node. This is called an ectopic atrial rhythm and unless particularly slow or fast, is a common, normal variant in children. P waves of different morphologies are called a wandering atrial pacemaker and is also a common normal variant in children.

Next is the PR interval that is measured from the beginning of the P wave to the beginning of the Q wave (not the R wave as the name suggests). Age-appropriate intervals for the PR have been established but generally do not exceed 200 ms. an abnormally prolonged PR interval usually indicates a problem in the AV node. Check for PR depression that may be a sign of myocarditis.

Next, turn to the QRS complexes and again, establish the rate of ventricular contractions, which should match the P wave rate. If this is not the case, it may be indicative of a significant rhythm change and possible electrophysiologic disease. Tall R

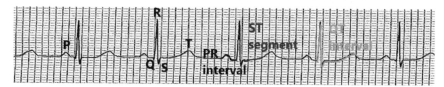

FIGURE 8.3 Waveforms and intervals/segments of an ECG.

Waveforms are identified by P, QRS, and T waves. Measured intervals include the PR (blue) and QT (green). Note that the PR interval is measured from the beginning of the P wave to the Q wave. The ST segment, which is part of the QT interval, may be elevated or depressed in relation to the ECG baseline during pathologic conditions (i.e., ischemia, inflammation, etc.).

waves can be indicative of ventricular hypertrophy while wide R waves could represent premature ventricular contractions or interventricular conduction delay such as bundle branch block. Establish the vector or axis of the QRS complexes (positive in I and aVF for normal conduction through the AV node).

Next, measure the QT interval from the beginning of the Q wave to the end of the T wave. Given the faster heart rate in children, the QT interval should be corrected (called the QTc) most commonly by Bazett's formula, QTc = QT interval (seconds) divided by the square root of the preceding R—R interval in seconds (see Fig. 8.4). This corrects the QT interval to a rate of 60 bpm. A prolonged QT may occur in hypokalemia and hypomagnesemia and as a result of certain medications, but often indicates a rare condition called Long QT Syndrome.

Abnormalities of the ST segment may indicate cardiac ischemia; however, so-called nonspecific ST segment elevation is a common normal finding in adolescents. Finally, T waves should be evaluated for a rate that should match the QRS complex rate as T waves represent the repolarization of the QRS depolarization of the ventricular myocardium. The presence of what appears to be additional T waves may actually be P waves as can be seen with atrial flutter or fibrillation. Tall T waves may suggest hyperkalemia. Broad or notched T waves may be seen in forms of Long QT syndrome. Lastly, the T wave vector or axis should be evaluated and should be consistent with QRS. Inverted T waves in lateral precordial leads (V4—V6) suggest left ventricular strain, and, when seen in combination with tall R waves, may be indicative of cardiomyopathy.

Pediatric electrocardiogram interpretation is a skill that is reinforced with every interpretation. A methodical approach is key to avoid making misinterpretations.

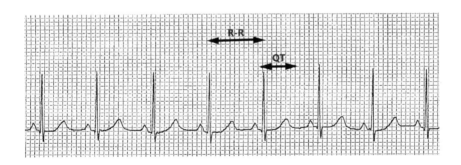

$$\text{Bazett's Formula QTc} = \frac{\text{QT interval (sec)}}{\sqrt{\text{R-R interval (sec)}}}$$

FIGURE 8.4 Calculation of QTc by Bazett's formula.

The purpose of corrected QT interval is to normalize to a heart rate of 60 bpm as heart rate influences the QT interval. The QT in seconds is divided by the square root of the preceding R—R interval in seconds.

Computer interpretations are often incorrect and any concerns should be properly assessed by a pediatric cardiologist or electrophysiologist.

Action plan

In the case of the child presenting to the pediatrician for a normal check-up and subsequently noted to have a low resting heart rate, the most likely diagnosis is sinus bradycardia that requires no further action other than continued observation. The diagnosis is established with the standard electrocardiogram. Abnormalities found on the electrocardiogram may prompt a more immediate response, often correlated with symptomatology. Consultation with pediatric cardiology is highly advised. In the scenario of heart block, treatment of reversible conditions (Lyme disease, myocarditis) should be immediately instituted while sustaining cardiac output with temporary pacing techniques. As with all heart rhythm related problems, treat the patient, not the electrocardiogram.

7-year-old presents to ER with recurrent SVT

Case

Sorry to bother you, I'm calling from the emergency room at Blank Regional Hospital, we're about 90 miles from your institution. We had a 7-year old female who has a history of supraventricular tachycardia (SVT) that presented with breakthrough tachycardia today at 220 bpm. I tried having her blow through an occluded straw and she was unable to break the tachycardia- this usually works for her. I was able to obtain an ECG and I am sending that to you now. I was going to give her adenosine 6 mg IV but the tachycardia broke as we were getting an IV. The reason I am calling you is that this is her fourth visit to the ER for this SVT. She was seen by a local adult cardiologist who had put her on a calcium channel blocker after her second visit, but it really hasn't worked. According to the mother, she is having breakthrough episodes nearly every day at school and they self-resolve after sitting in the nurse's office for about 30 minutes. They were told that anything longer she should seek medical attention. Her dose on the calcium channel blocker is pretty good for her weight and she has had some significant constipation issues with it. I'm wondering if I should try a different medication or have her come see you?

What am I thinking?

Whenever I hear a story like this, I am often left wondering *why I haven't seen this child sooner*? The rate of 220 and the ability to break with vagal maneuvers are very consistent with a reentrant tachycardia that is AV nodal dependent. Atrioventricular reentrant tachycardia is the most likely secondary to an accessory pathway given her age. Having breakthrough tachycardia daily is unacceptable, especially at this age. My inclination is to have a visit with the family and seriously discuss the option of catheter ablation, or a trial of a different medication.

Arrhythmias in Children. https://doi.org/10.1016/B978-0-323-77907-4.00009-3

Differential diagnosis
Likely
Atrioventricular reentrant tachycardia (AVRT), accessory pathway mediated Atrioventricular nodal reentrant tachycardia (AVNRT)
Possible
Ventricular tachycardia, outflow tract
Rare
Ectopic atrial tachycardia

History and physical

In the child or adolescent who is having recurrent arrhythmias, an arrhythmia history can be very helpful in guiding treatment and understanding potential mechanisms. For the child with SVT, the sensation can be difficult to explain and is often expressed in their imaginative way. Children may state that their heart is "running" or "beeping" very fast. Some may simply complain that their "heart hurts" given limited ability to express tachycardia and not reflecting true angina. Children are usually quite perceptive of the sudden onset of tachycardia though the sudden offset is less recognized. They are often quite clear when they are in tachycardia and when they are not. Common complaints associated with tachycardia is the feeling of light-headedness or dizziness, shortness of breath, and all accompanied by the feeling that the heart is "beating out" of the chest. Some express the feeling of nausea and on occasion chest discomfort, though not often found to have true cardiac chest pain. Rarely do children present with syncope and this may warrant further workup for other arrhythmias or inherited arrhythmia syndromes. Family members will often say that the child does not look right during the episode, usually appearing slightly pale and "out of it." Smaller children often choose to stop involvement in activities and wish to rest. Older children are quite clear that something feels off and left to their own devices, will look to rest.

Attention is often turned to triggers the start of the tachycardia. Most commonly physical activity is a trigger for reentrant tachycardias. This may be a result of alterations in the AV nodal conduction and refractory zones or an increase in ectopic beats. Often, older children will complain that when they are participating in physical education or playing sports, they note the SVT. In such instances, we often advise that they should discontinue actively playing and attempt to break the tachycardia on the sidelines. Once the tachycardia has ceased, return to activity is allowed after approximately 10 min of rest.

For some, a trigger may be dietary and related to caffeine intake such as in sodas, coffees, or energy drinks. Caffeine can increase the frequency of ectopic beats such as premature atrial and premature ventricular beats. This increase in ectopy can lead to frequent tachycardias. Understanding potential triggers can help in planning for electrophysiology study and needs for induction of tachycardia (e.g., use of beta-agonist such as isoproterenol). Physical examination is primarily focused on the determination of an associated structural heart problem; however, this is uncommon.

For patients who are considered candidates for electrophysiology study and ablation, there are aspects of the history and physical that should be ascertained. It is wise to ask about the family history regarding any bleeding disorders or bleeding tendencies (i.e., von Willebrand, heparin-induced thrombocytopenia), likewise clotting disorders or clotting tendencies (i.e., Factor V Leiden). Most studies in the young are performed under general anesthesia, asking for family or personal history of anesthesia reactions including malignant hyperthermia. Asking family about other members who have undergone a cardiac ablation or catheterization can help to gauge their understanding of the procedure. Determining other past medical histories such as diabetes or asthma can also help with planning. Patients will need to fast before the procedure and special care has to be taken in diabetics to manage their blood sugar appropriately. Adenosine, which is often used in the procedure, can induce significant bronchospasm in some patients with asthma and the anesthesiologist should be alerted before administration. As intubation is required for general anesthesia, knowing about loose teeth or any neck deformities is best known ahead of time. From a physical examination standpoint, the focus should be on clearly understanding vascular access points and if there are any obstructions such as the previous history of femoral catheterization or central line placement. Additionally, those patients who suffer from physical disabilities may have significant issues with lying on a table supine for several hours or may have contractures that prevent proper positioning.

Diagnostic testing

For patients preparing for an electrophysiology study and ablation, several tests can provide critical information. The first is the electrocardiogram at baseline to determine if ventricular preexcitation is present (see Figs. 13.1 and 13.2). An electrocardiogram of the tachycardia will also be helpful as certain appearances can indicate mechanism and pathway location. If the onset and offset were able to have been caught on an electrocardiogram or monitor strip, this can also be very helpful.

An echocardiogram is necessary to determine the cardiac anatomy and assessment of cardiac function. Special attention should also be focused on vascular abnormalities such as an interrupted inferior vena cava or left superior vena cava to the coronary sinus. The finding of an atrial communication may also influence decisions regarding the transseptal approach and timing of heparinization during the procedure.

If there are any questions regarding vascular patency due to prior history of cannulation, a vascular study should be performed before the procedure to verify. For female patients who have the potential for pregnancy, a pregnancy test must be ordered given the radiation exposure with fluoroscopy.

Action plan

The decision to proceed with an electrophysiology study and catheter ablation can be a difficult one for families. The Pediatric and Congenital Electrophysiology Society along with the Heart Rhythm Society has published comprehensive and thorough guidelines regarding indications for ablation in children. Generally, patients who are at least 15 kg and ages 7–8 years who are experiencing recurrent tachycardia that is either refractory to medical therapies, results in ventricular dysfunction, or requires frequent emergency room visits are considered good candidates for ablation with safe and effective outcomes.

When discussing the treatment of the standard narrow complex SVT child, there are several options presented to the parents. The first is to continue to monitor without intervention. This is usually reserved for the child who has a rare occurrence of SVT (say once per year) that is short in duration or can be easily broken without the need for medical services. The second option is to initiate and modify medications for those patients that have recurrent SVT. First line agents can include digoxin, β-blockers, or calcium channel blockers and various combinations of the three. Sodium channel blockers and class III agents are generally felt to be the second line. The risks of medications include potential side effects as well as the need for compliance with at least daily and often multiple doses per day. The benefit is that the patient can avoid a procedure, and in some cases, can avoid any further SVT with a medication taken once daily.

Finally, the option of catheter ablation for children who have multiple recurrences of SVT who may be refractory to medications or wish to have a more permanent solution to their tachycardia. Patients are brought to the cardiac catheterization lab where fluoroscopy equipment can be used to guide catheters to the heart. With three-dimensional mapping systems, the modern era of ablation has entered a low to zero-fluoroscopy model, minimizing the amount of radiation to the patient. As was mentioned previously, most electrophysiology studies and ablations are performed under general anesthesia or deep sedation in children. The patient is prepped and draped in a sterile fashion.

Access is obtained in various vascular structures, usually the femoral veins bilaterally. Right internal jugular and femoral arterial access may be obtained. Using a modified Seldinger technique, sheaths of various sizes are placed in the access locations to be able to place and exchange catheters that are long, coated wires that contain electrodes at the distal tip capable of recording the local electrical activity at the adjacent cardiac tissue. Electrical potentials can also be sent through the catheter to activate the adjacent cardiac tissue or "pace" the heart leading to a cardiac contraction. These catheters are placed into various positions of the heart to obtain signals from structures such as the sinus node (high right atrial catheter), atrioventricular node (His catheter), ventricle (right ventricle catheter), and the mitral valve annulus (coronary sinus catheter) (see Fig. 9.1). With catheters in place, an electrophysiology study is performed using various diagnostic techniques involving pacing to understand the baseline electrical system and induction of arrhythmia. Based on the pattern of activation and other diagnostic maneuvers, the mechanism of arrhythmia can be deduced (see Figs. 9.2 and 9.3).

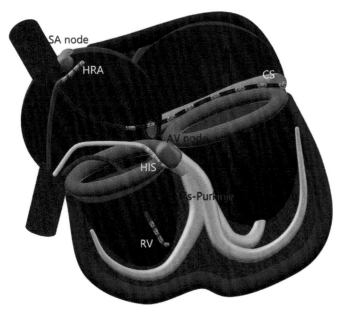

FIGURE 9.1 Catheter locations for standard pediatric electrophysiology study.

Catheter placement locations are based on the cardiac conduction system. The high right atrium catheter (HRA) (orange catheter) is placed near the sino-atrial (SA) node. The SA node is located at the junction of the superior vena cava and right atrium (depicted in gold). The HIS catheter (green) is intended to reflect the activity of the atrioventricular (AV) node and the His bundle, located at the junction between the atria and ventricles (depicted in gold). The His bundle is located anteriorly on the tricuspid valve and provides a characteristic, sharp electrogram between the atrial and ventricular electrogram. The His-Purkinje system (yellow) is what transmits the depolarization from the AV node into rapid ventricular activation. Typically, a right ventricular (RV) (pink) catheter is placed to provide ventricular activation and act as a pacing site if required. Lastly, a coronary sinus catheter (CS) (blue) is placed into the coronary sinus and runs posteriorly along the mitral valve annulus and provides activation information on the left side of the heart. The electrophysiologist uses these catheter placements to create a map of the electrical activation sequence in the heart.

The next step in the procedure is the mapping of the arrhythmia to the substrate and the use of cardiac ablation to eliminate the substrate. Using a variety of techniques, the substrate of the arrhythmia is mapped to a location within the heart. In the event of an accessory pathway-mediated tachycardia, the location of the accessory pathway is identified along the tricuspid or mitral valves. In the case of the mitral valve, access must be obtained to the left side of the heart that may be performed via transseptal procedure or using a retrograde approach through the arterial access with preference left to the pediatric electrophysiologist. A separate catheter is used for precise mapping and delivery of energy to ablate the substrate. There are

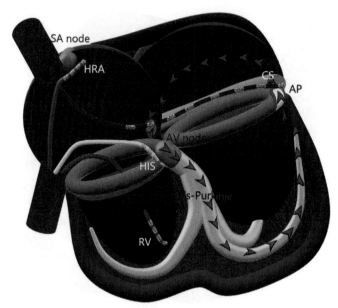

FIGURE 9.2 Depiction of left-sided accessory pathway-mediated tachycardia.

A left-sided accessory pathway (AP) bridges the left atrium and left ventricle along the mitral valve annulus (depicted in yellow with red border). The circuit for supraventricular tachycardia depicted is orthodromic: meaning that conduction is antegrade through the AV node, through the His-Purkinje system, and traverses the accessory pathway back into the left atrium to complete the circuit (red arrowheads). The site of the earliest atrial activation after ventricular activation in this arrhythmia serves as the atrial insertion site of the accessory pathway. Delivery of ablation energy to this location would eliminate pathway conduction and thereby terminate tachycardia by eliminating the circuit.

two forms of ablation energy used in the current era of pediatric ablation, cryothermal energy and radiofrequency energy. Using a specific catheter for the specified energy source, this energy is applied to a discrete area of ablation at the catheter tip that destroys the cells at that location thereby eliminating the substrate. Success for ablation in children for typical SVT is estimated to be around 95%. By eliminating the substrate, the arrhythmia can no longer be supported and the patient is essentially cured of the condition with a low risk of recurrence. Procedure time can vary but is on average about 4–5 h. There are no incisions, no stitches, and patients can often go home the same day with the resumption of full activities within 1 week.

As with any procedure, there are risks involved though quite minimal. As access is being obtained, there is the risk of bleeding or infection. It is not uncommon for patients to have bruising or development of a hematoma at the access site. Other complications of procedural access include vascular complications, perforation of

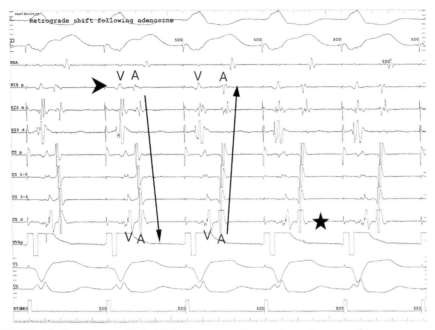

FIGURE 9.3 Electrogram of left-sided accessory pathway retrograde conduction.

Figure is taken from an electrophysiology study of a concealed left-sided accessory pathway. Ventricular electrogram is marked with a "V" and atrial electrogram is marked with an "A." Ventricular pacing is performed every 500 ms and demonstrates retrograde conduction through the AV node with first atrial activation at the level of His (arrowhead) and followed by CS proximal (CSp) to CS distal (CSd). During ventricular pacing, adenosine is administered, which blocks conduction in the AV node, changing the retrograde conduction pattern with earliest atrial activation at the site of the pathway on the left side (star). Here, CS distal has the earliest atrial activation followed by CS proximal with atrial activation later in the His.

blood vessels or the heart, which are very rare. With a catheter in place, there is the risk of arrhythmias, thrombus formation, and damage to surrounding structures such as cardiac valves or coronary arteries, which are also very rare. The most significant risk for cardiac ablation in children is the risk of damage to the AV node that would result in the need for a pacemaker and is estimated to be a risk of approximately 1%. Major complications such as radiation injury, stroke, pulmonary embolism, myocardial infarction, or death are much less than 1%.

Electrophysiology study and cardiac ablation in children is safe and effective. With all procedures, an open and honest discussion about the risks and benefits is vital to have an informed choice from the family and the patient. While anxiety and fear are common, it can be addressed with clear communication and answering questions that parents and patients may have. Outcomes of catheter ablation can be life-changing for patients by providing a cure to their recurrent arrhythmias.

Suggested reading

Philip Saul J, Kanter RJ, Writing Committee, et al. PACES/HRS expert consensus statement on the use of catheter ablation in children and patients with congenital heart disease: developed in partnership with the Pediatric and Congenital Electrophysiology Society (PACES) and the Heart Rhythm Society (HRS). Endorsed by the governing bodies of PACES, HRS, the American Academy of Pediatrics (AAP), the American Heart Association (AHA), and the Association for European Pediatric and Congenital Cardiology (AEPC). *Heart Rhythm.* 2016;13(6):e251−e289. https://doi.org/10.1016/j.hrthm.2016.02.009.

6-year-old presents with mildly elevated heart rate that is persistent

Case

Hi, thanks for taking my call. I have a 6-year old female who presents today for what appears to be an otitis media on her right ear. Mom says she has had a day of fever and has been complaining of ear pain. The reason I am calling is that when she came into the office, her heart rate was 150 bpm. She had a temperature of 39.5°C at the time, so I thought maybe it was related to the fever. I had the mom give her a dose of acetaminophen and a few hours later had them come back for a heart rate check and it remains at 150 bpm with a normal temperature. I'm honestly not sure what to make of this heart rate. She appears asymptomatic except for her ear but the heart rate worries me. Anything I should do about it?

What am I thinking?

I am impressed by the pediatrician's efforts to investigate an anomaly rather than excuse it. While a fever can certainly increase heart rate, a heart rate of 150 bpm for a 6-year old female is higher than would be expected. Rather than excuse the heart rate as a normal variant, the pediatrician appropriately treats the fever and asks that the patient return for follow-up demonstrating that the heart rate remains elevated. From this point, I begin to consider arrhythmia in the differential as to why this patient is tachycardic. Sinus tachycardia may have occurred for other reasons outside of fever, but my first thoughts are to help identify the rhythm using an electrocardiogram and long-term monitoring for determianation of the persistence of the rate. From there, an assessment of cardiac function may be performed to rule-out a tachycardia-induced cardiomyopathy.

Arrhythmias in Children. https://doi.org/10.1016/B978-0-323-77907-4.00010-X

Differential diagnosis
Likely
Ectopic atrial tachycardia, multifocal atrial tachycardia
Persistent junctional reciprocating tachycardia
Possible
Ventricular tachycardia
Rare
Myocarditis leading to arrhythmia
Sinus tachycardia due to thyrotoxicosis
Sinus tachycardia due to pheochromocytoma

History and physical

Assessment of the patient with a persistent arrhythmia should focus on identification of the rhythm and hemodynamic consequences of said rhythm. In most cases, the patient is young and cannot identify the timing of the arrhythmia initiation or cessation. In cases where patients may be able to better communicate, using colloquial language to discuss arrhythmias may be helpful. Pediatric patients can use creative language to describe the feeling of palpitations including "heart beeping" or "heart flashing." Sometimes children will describe a sensation of palpitations as "pain" (i.e., "my heart hurts"). It should be noted that chest pain in pediatrics is relatively common and may not necessarily reflect arrhythmia but should be considered in the differential.

Additional symptoms should be elicited from family members and caretakers. Those patients who begin to have tachycardia-induced cardiomyopathy symptoms may describe a decrease in physical activity or an inability to keep up with other children. An increased propensity for taking naps compared to prior habits may be a sign of fatigue. In severe cases, patients may have more telling features of congestive heart failure such as respiratory distress due to pulmonary edema, nausea and/or vomiting, and poor growth. Recent ill contacts or recent respiratory illnesses may provide clues to a developing myocarditis. Review any new medications or supplements that may be in use.

Assessment of vital signs for elevated respiratory rate, decreased pulse oximetry, elevated heart rate, or reduced blood pressure would be concerning for cardiomyopathy. Fever may be suggestive of an infectious etiology as in myocarditis. On examination, cardiac auscultation should reveal an elevated heart rate and possibly an irregular rhythm due to ectopic beats. In severe cardiomyopathy, an S3 or S4 gallop may be present though an S3 gallop may be a normal finding in children. A murmur could be present as a result of valvular regurgitation (i.e., mitral valve regurgitation). Evidence of hepatosplenomegaly and peripheral edema are also signs of congestive heart failure. Assessment of the child's breathing pattern and listening for crackles suggestive of pulmonary edema help complete the clinical picture.

Diagnostic testing

The first test for assessment of the rhythm is an electrocardiogram. If the rhythm is persistent or frequent, it is possible that an ECG and rhythm strip may be able to capture the necessary information. In those cases where the rhythm occurs intermittently, a Holter (or other ambulatory) monitor may be necessary but such rhythms are unlikely to result in a cardiomyopathy. An echocardiogram should be considered to assess cardiac function. If an arrhythmia is noted, other lab work may be indicated such as evaluation for electrolyte abnormalities or thyroid testing. Other lab testing may be beneficial if ruling out rare diseases such as a pheochromocytoma where urine catecholamines may be diagnostic.

Action plan

Patient stability is the primary action. This usually involves hospitalization for the management of any heart failure symptoms for those who have decompensated due to the arrhythmia. Appropriate treatment for electrolyte abnormalities or the use of diuretics may be helpful in the immediate term. Inotropic (improved systolic function) and lusitropic (improves diastolic function) medications may be utilized for those with severely depressed function but deserve a word of caution as these agents may also be proarrhythmic. In the significantly compromised patient, other supportive measures may be required including the use of ventricular assistance utilizing extracorporeal membrane oxygenation. With hemodynamic stability, attention is turned immediately to rhythm control.

Depending on the suspected etiology and age of the patient, electrophysiology study and potential ablation can be diagnostic and therapeutic. This is particularly true for persistent junctional reciprocating tachycardia (see Fig. 10.1), which is a reentrant form of arrhythmia secondary to an accessory pathway most often located in the posterior septal region of the tricuspid valve annulus. This form of the accessory pathway has decremental conduction properties resulting in an easily sustainable arrhythmia (see Fig. 10.2). Ablation of the pathway eliminates the substrate for arrhythmia and cures the patient of further arrhythmia allowing for recovery of ventricular function. This has become the gold standard of treatment in most patients unless there are significant concerns for harm by ablation such as in very small children. Medications are considered less optimal, and patients often need treatment with strong antiarrhythmics from the sodium channel blocker or potassium channel blocker groups.

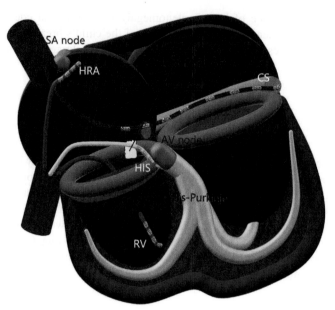

FIGURE 10.1 Anatomic location of AP in PJRT.

The typical location of the accessory pathway (AP) that leads to persistent junctional reciprocating tachycardia (PJRT) is posterior septal to posterior along the tricuspid valve. The pathway (depicted in yellow with red border) has decremental conduction similar to the AV node that allows for tachycardia persistence. *AP*, accessory pathway; *AV*, atrioventricular; *CS*, coronary sinus catheter; *HIS*, His bundle catheter; *HRA*, high right atrium catheter; *RV*, Right ventricular catheter; *SA*, Sinoatria.

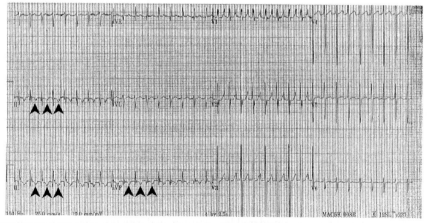

FIGURE 10.2 Persistent junctional reciprocating tachycardia.

ECG of an infant with a long RP tachycardia demonstrating P waves that are negative in leads II, III, and aVF (arrowheads) consistent with a persistent junctional reciprocating tachycardia. Ectopic atrial tachycardia is also in the differential. The patient underwent catheter ablation of a posterior septal accessory pathway consistent with persistent junctional reciprocating tachycardia.

Patients with atrial tachycardia are a bit more challenging but are usually suscep-tible to ablation for the elimination of their substrate. These forms of tachycardia are regionalized to a group of ectopic cells within the atria that create an automatic rhythm opposing that of sinus rhythm. This ectopic focus can be ablated utilizing the timing of arrhythmia combined with a three-dimensional mapping system to identify the earliest activation, which is the target.

In the setting of multifocal atrial tachycardia, the substrate originates in multiple areas that may not be easily amenable to ablation. Multifocal atrial tachycardia often requires medications for management. Drug challenges during EP study may pro-vide some insights as to which agents to utilize or perform medication optimization during an inpatient hospitalization with telemetry monitoring. Given the automa-ticity of the arrhythmia, medication choices usually revolve around agents with sodium or potassium channel blocking activity. These medications can have side ef-fects and proarrhythmic effects that must be monitored, particularly in the young. Most initial doses or significant medication adjustments are performed inpatient with a pediatric cardiologist or electrophysiologist.

8-year-old presents with ADHD presents to cardiology office with ECG in hand for "cardiac clearance" to start stimulants

11

Case

Hi doctor, this is the check-in desk calling from the waiting room. I have a mother here who has brought her 8-year old son with an electrocardiogram (ECG) in her hands stating that she needs to have this read before she can get a prescription for ADHD medications. You have never seen this child before, but the mother is insisting that the ECG be read today as the child is starting back at school next week. She says her pediatrician won't allow her to get the prescription unless a cardiologist clears him. I've tried to get her to schedule an appointment, but she keeps insisting that all she needs is the ECG to be read by someone to clear her son for stimulant medications. Does this sound like something you can do?

What am I thinking?

To be honest, I am as frustrated as the mother. ECG screening is a controversial topic for a variety of reasons. While seemingly simple, the questions posed raise a number of complex issues. Like many tests, the ECG has strengths and limitations when it comes to providing answers to the type of question posed by this mother. Sometimes it can give a specific answer, but often, it may raise issues well beyond the question for which it was performed. Hence, one needs to be cautious, and not take the matter too lightly. Without understanding the context of the ECG, it can provide false reassurance or send the physician down a deep rabbit hole of tests with no clear end in sight. Therefore, to use an often misused and overused dictum: "Clinical correlation is always advised and necessary." Which is to say that the context is key. (*Continued at end of chapter*).

Arrhythmias in Children. https://doi.org/10.1016/B978-0-323-77907-4.00011-1

Conditions that can lead to sudden cardiac arrest diagnosed by ECG in the asymptomatic child

Likely
Pre-excitation syndromes (Wolff-Parkinson-White)
Possible
Long QT Syndrome Short QT Syndrome Hypertrophic Cardiomyopathy Dilated cardiomyopathy Aortic stenosis
Rare
Brugada Syndrome Arrhythmogenic Right Ventricular Cardiomyopathy Marfan Syndrome
Unlikely/Normal baseline ECG
Anomalous Coronary Artery Catecholaminergic Polymorphic Ventricular Tachycardia Idiopathic Ventricular Fibrillation

History and physical

In the scenario presented, there would not be an opportunity to perform a thorough history and physician without an appointment. However, the purpose of this section is to highlight cardiac screening in the young and the type of evaluation it involves. The American Academy of Pediatrics has a preparticipation physical evaluation that includes a helpful history screening questions in the heart health section of the form. While the questions are purposefully somewhat vague, "yes" answers to the questions may prompt more questions and further evaluation.

Have you ever passed out or nearly passed out during or after exercise?

Syncope during exercise is concerning for both structural and arrhythmic diagnoses for sudden cardiac death. Further questions into the timing of syncope, the circumstances, emergency response, etc. will be crucial in determining if this patient may have a condition that may be potentially lethal and associated with sudden death. Most structural heart disease and inherited arrhythmia syndromes can present as syncope with exercise, and this one symptom should always be taken very seriously and be considered an aborted sudden death episode until otherwise disproven.

Have you ever had discomfort, pain, tightness or pressure in your chest during exercise?

The key to this question is during exercise. Chest pain is a common complaint in young people and adolescents, usually occurring at rest and can be reproduced on physical exam. However, when present during exercise, chest pain should be considered a symptom pointing to a serious heart condition like coronary ischemia, which, in children, can be caused by conditions such as anomalous origin or course of the coronary artery, hypertrophic cardiomyopathy, and dilated cardiomyopathy.

Does your heart ever race, flutter in your chest, or skip beats (irregular beats) during exercise?

This question is attempting to identify conditions in which exercise may predispose to an arrhythmia such as Wolff-Parkinson-White Syndrome, Hypertrophic Cardiomyopathy (HCM), Arrhythmogenic Right Ventricular Dysplasia (ARVD), and Catecholaminergic Polymorphic Ventricular Tachycardia (CPVT). This question is particularly important for CPVT as an increased catecholamine state is what predisposes to arrhythmia in CPVT. Also, CPVT patients may sometimes have PVCs on the ECG, but it is not uncommon for the ECG (and physical examination) to be normal in these patients. Patients can be diagnosed by exercise stress test with a pathognomonic pattern of bidirectional ventricular tachycardia (Reference to Chapter 18, Figure 1).

Has a doctor ever told you that you have any heart problems?; Has a doctor ever requested a test for your heart? For example, electrocardiography (ECG) or echocardiography?

These questions are driving toward patients who have been diagnosed with either congenital or acquired heart disease and require further evaluation for physical activity by their cardiologists. Patients who mark yes to these questions should be assessed by a cardiologist and may indeed require further testing to assess fitness for physical activity.

Do you get light-headed or feel short of breath earlier than your friends during exercise?

This question is attempting to determine whether the stress of exercise can unmask an underlying serious heart condition and on the heart's ability to compensate for exercise. In patients with structural heart disease, this can manifest as feeling light-headed or becoming short of breath faster than peers. This may be true in patients with hypertrophic cardiomyopathy or anomalous origin of the coronary artery and maybe the first sign of a cardiac problem.

Have you ever had a seizure?

While seizure activity is certainly a concern of neurologic conditions, the question is posed in the cardiac health history to determine any prior presentation of cardiac arrest lading to cerebral anoxia that, in turn, can cause a seizure. This is particularly helpful in assessing arrhythmia-related diseases (such as long QT syndrome, short QT syndrome, Brugada syndrome, ARVD, and CPVT) where, for poorly understood reasons, arrhythmias can be nonsustained and self-terminate. Thus, the patient can have recurrent "seizures" and can be mistakenly treated for epilepsy. Other cardiac conditions that may present with arrhythmic arrest can also be manifest with seizure-like activity. For patients who do have a history of seizure, it is helpful to further define their neurologic workup and whether a seizure disorder was diagnosed or remains unexplained.

Screening questions then turn to family history. For genetic arrhythmia syndromes, family history is critical to help establish the need for further testing and diagnosis. When assessing a child for inherited syndromes, take the time to perform a thorough and detailed family history. Simply put it can be lifesaving, not only for the patient, but for other family members as well.

Has any family member or relative died of heart problems or had an unexpected or unexplained sudden death before age 35 years (including drowning or unexplained car crash)? Has anyone in your family had a pacemaker or an implanted defibrillator before age 35?

These questions are attempting to tease out the possibility of acquired heart disease or coronary artery disease by using an age cut-off of 35 years. Coronary artery disease due to atherosclerosis is such a common problem in older persons and relatively uncommon below 35. This is not to say that coronary artery disease cannot manifest before the age of 35 years; only that it is less common. Hence, a sudden or unexplained death in a relatively young person (<35) should lead to an extensive search for conditions such as HCM, abnormal coronary arteries, and channelopathies. Unexplained or unexpected sudden death should be further investigated to determine the circumstances around the event and the health condition of the deceased before the event. For example, a car accident occurring at 10 a.m. due to collision with a truck on the highway resulting in death of the passenger is very different from an individual driving alone at 10 a.m. who suddenly crosses lanes and suffers a head-on collision with a vehicle traveling the opposite direction with the latter suggesting a cardiac event while driving. Another example would a person who knew how to swim ending up drowning in a swimming pool. Family members who have required the need of a pacemaker or defibrillator below the age of 35 may be a sign of genetic arrhythmia syndromes. As most genetic syndromes are inherited in an autosomal dominant fashion, identification of the relationship to the patient and other potentially affected family members is also critical to the investigation. A family pedigree is created to assess family member risks and inheritance patterns during genetic counseling.

Does anyone in your family have a genetic heart problem such as hypertrophic cardiomyopathy, Marfan syndrome, arrhythmogenic right ventricular cardiomyopathy, long QT syndrome, short QT syndrome, Brugada syndrome, or catecholaminergic polymorphic ventricular tachycardia?

Clearly this question is seeking to identify specific diagnoses in family members. It is important to use these terms and synonymous terms in obtaining a history. Many of these conditions by name are difficult to relate to the cardiac system for the average person. As such, they may recall that a family member has a condition but not necessarily relate that this is cardiac related. Additionally, describing some of the conditions can help patients provide a better history such as describing hypertrophic cardiomyopathy as a "thickened" heart. Sometimes understanding what form of work-up was pursued may help patients reveal conditions in family members that can lead the interviewer down the correct path toward diagnosis.

Turning to the physical examination, the examiner is encouraged to utilize a full examination for the detection of potential cardiac disease. While this has traditionally focused on auscultation, other signs of cardiac disease may be demonstrable on examination. Marfan syndrome or other connective tissue disorders that may result in aortic dissection have specific features that may aide in diagnosis. The revised Ghent nosology is used for Marfan Syndrome in combination of family history, aortic dilation, and ectopia lentis. A hyperactive precordium or presence of a thrill may be discovered by palpation of the chest and may signal the presence of structural heart disease. The murmur of aortic stenosis and hypertrophic cardiomyopathy is systolic. Use of diagnostic maneuvers while auscultating can help distinguish and are directly related to preload and afterload of the heart. Asking the patient to move from a standing to squatting position increases the preload that results in a louder murmur for aortic stenosis but softens the murmur for hypertrophic cardiomyopathy. A return to standing reduces the preload and increases the intensity of the murmur of hypertrophic cardiomyopathy while reducing the murmur for aortic stenosis. Similarly, Valsalva maneuver also reduces the preload and results in the same changes to murmur as standing.

Diagnostic testing

In the scenario presented, the patient and mother came to the office with an ECG in hand. For this section, the debate of the screening ECG will be briefly discussed. The screening ECG is controversial in the pediatric electrophysiology community sparking numerous, passionate debates and position papers. As mentioned in previous chapters, the ECG is an excellent tool for the evaluation of rhythm related disorders in symptomatic patients. It is not a first-choice test for the evaluation of structural heart disease. But the simplicity of obtaining and low cost, make it appealing for an initial evaluation. By definition, the screening ECG is performed in the asymptomatic patient without prior history or concern of familial or personal cardiac disease. For certain disease such as Wolff-Parkinson-White, the resting ECG is diagnostic while for others such as CPVT, it is of little to no use. Much has been written on the probability of sudden death prevention with the use of screening ECG versus history/physical alone. There is little debate on the increase of pretest probability and reliability of a combined approach.

The challenge is not at the level of the individual, but at the level of public health. Are screening ECGs the best method to determine the likelihood of sudden death in the young? Once completed, the ECG must be correctly interpreted that can raise some complexity. Further points of debate include who needs an ECG? Athletes? Nonathletes? School-aged children? Newborns? Should it be repeated? How often? Are screening ECGs the most cost-effective method? How does this impact communities with lower socioeconomic status? Could public health dollars be better spent to affect the overall health of the public? These questions and more spark intense debate on the subject. While debate continues among experts, the lack of consensus has led to a localized or regionalized approach to screening ECGs.

Action plan

A few words on the terminology of "cardiac clearance." Clearance may imply that the cardiologist or electrophysiologist has determined that the patient may undergo a procedure or start a medication based on the cardiac evaluation. A more appropriate definition is that the cardiologist or electrophysiologist has evaluated the patient from a cardiac perspective and feels that the benefit of the procedure or medication outweighs the cardiovascular risk at this time. The term "clearance" may suggest the elimination of risk, but this is most certainly not the case.

ECG screening in the pediatric patient considering stimulant medications for attention deficit disorders has a complicated and controversial history that will briefly be reviewed. Initial case reports of adverse events related to long-term use of methylphenidate including acute myocardial infarction and cardiac arrest in two adolescents prompted concern with stimulant use and cardiovascular effects. The Food and Drug Administration's (FDA) adverse event reporting system recorded 11 cases of sudden death among pediatric patients on methylphenidate from January 1992 to February 2005 prompting the agency to place a warning label on amphetamine mixed salts in August of 2005. The issue was further escalated by the FDA to a black-box warning in February 2006. In 2007, the FDA recommended that drug manufactures prepare patient medication guidelines and alert them of cardiovascular risk and sudden death in those with preexisting heart conditions. This was followed in 2008 by a recommendation for screening ECGs by the American Heart Association that was soon followed by a rebuttal by the American Academy of Pediatrics.

What has not been debated are the effects of stimulant medication, resulting in a mild increase in heart rate and blood pressure that are well-tolerated in the normal population. The concern relates to those medication-induced changes in a more vulnerable population, specifically those with underlying cardiac disease. To date, there have been no long-term, controlled studies evaluating the cardiovascular risk for patients with and without cardiovascular disease. This reverts to the discussion on appropriate screening methodology for asymptomatic cardiac disease and use of the ECG to properly weigh the risks and benefits of proposed change.

A few facts have been certain and receive general consensus: (1) Patients with known cardiac disease should be under the consultation and follow-up of a pediatric cardiologist before initiating stimulant and stimulant-like medications; (2) Patients with concerning history or physical examination findings suggestive of cardiac disease should undergo consultation with a pediatric cardiologist before initiating new medication or new activity; (3) Patients with concerns for cardiac arrhythmia or sudden arrhythmic death should undergo an ECG; (4) A resting ECG can be both diagnostic and nondiagnostic depending on the sudden cardiac death condition investigated; (5) ECG interpretation is a skill that must be developed and should never be left to current ECG machine interpretation alone.

What am I thinking? (*Continued*)

Given the above information, I would ask the pediatrician to not just look at the ECG but also get a history and examination as described. I would also offer to review the ECG and ask them to send it to me via facsimile or other means.

If the ECG is completely normal in my opinion, I would pass that on and tell the pediatrician that this is a reassuring ECG. As long as the mother understands that there can be false negative ECGs (patient has a condition but the ECG looks normal), the child can be allowed to take ADHD medications.

If the ECG shows abnormal or borderline findings (nonspecific or questionable findings that do not clearly point to a certain condition yet are concerning), the patient needs to have an outpatient visit with a pediatric cardiologist before ADHD medications can be considered appropriate for him. The final decision whether to start medications may end up being a complex discussion between the cardiologist, pediatrician, and family to make sure that risks and benefits have been thoroughly weighed.

Suggested readings

AAP.org. *Preparticipation physical evaluation (PPE)*; 2020. Available at: https://www.aap.org/en-us/advocacy-and-policy/aap-health-initiatives/Pages/PPE.aspx. Accessed November 16, 2020.

American Academy of Pediatrics/American Heart Association. American Academy of Pediatrics/American Heart Association clarification of statement on cardiovascular evaluation and monitoring of children and adolescents with heart disease receiving medications for ADHD: May 16, 2008. *J Dev Behav Pediatr.* 2008;29(4):335. https://doi.org/10.1097/DBP.0b013e31318185dc14.

Cooper WO, Habel LA, Sox CM, et al. ADHD drugs and serious cardiovascular events in children and young adults. *N Engl J Med.* 2011;365(20):1896−1904. https://doi.org/10.1056/NEJMoa1110212.

Shahani SA, Evans WN, Mayman GA, Thomas VC. Attention deficit hyperactivity disorder screening electrocardiograms: a community-based perspective. *Pediatr Cardiol.* 2014; 35(3):485−489. https://doi.org/10.1007/s00246-013-0810-5.

11-year-old whose father recently died at the age of 40

Case

Thank you for taking my call. I am a local pediatrician and I just had a mother come in with her son for an evaluation. He is an 11-year old young man who I have been following since birth and has no real medical history to speak about. But the reason I am calling you is that the mother informed me today that his father had passed, suddenly, 2 weeks ago, at the age of forty. According to mom, the father had no previous medical history and so all of this is a complete shock. The family is saying he had some kind of "heart attack" but he never had any cardiac history prior and from what I saw of him, he was fit and healthy. Someone from the family has a background in medicine and suggested that the child be evaluated for the risk of sudden death. The mother is obviously devastated and fearful for her son's life. I'm wondering if there is anything special, I should be doing?

What am I thinking?

It is always difficult to manage the sudden loss of a family member. There is a balance in affording the family the appropriate time to grieve while ensuring that the appropriate actions be taken to provide much needed answers to this tragedy. Given the sudden nature of the death and the relatively young age of the parent, it raises concerns about the potential for an inherited cardiomyopathy or arrhythmic syndrome that may put first-degree relatives at risk. Any details surrounding the father's medical history or symptomatology will be important to elicit as well as the circumstances around the death. It will also be important to determine if an autopsy was performed or if this was a coroner's case that may also help provide clues as to the condition that led to the sudden death. Finally, obtaining blood samples from the deceased, which must be preserved in a purple top tube and can be frozen for future genetic testing can be critical for further diagnostic testing of family members. These conversations are difficult with grieving family members but many times, they can help to determine appropriate next steps and help provide some answers to the ultimate question of *"why did this happen?"*.

Arrhythmias in Children. https://doi.org/10.1016/B978-0-323-77907-4.00012-3

Inheritable primary cardiac conditions that can lead to sudden death
Hypertrophic cardiomyopathy
Long QT syndrome
Dilated cardiomyopathy
Arrhythmogenic ventricular dysplasia/cardiomyopathy
Brugada syndrome
Catecholaminergic polymorphic ventricular tachycardia
Short QT syndrome

History and physical

Any child with a first-degree relative who suffers a sudden unexplained death before the age of 35 (some publications consider before the age of 50) with possible cardiac origin should be evaluated by a pediatric cardiologist. As part of that evaluation, a thorough cardiac history of the child should be obtained to determine if there are any signs and/or symptoms suggestive of cardiac disease. A physical examination should also be completed with attention to any pathologic murmurs.

Next, the history must turn to the family member who suffered a sudden cardiac arrest. This can be a very painful time for the family and questions should be asked with the utmost level of sensitivity to the situation. It is important to ascertain the prior health of the deceased, specifically asking about diagnosed medical conditions, medications taken, and unexplained syncopal or seizure events. Directly ask about any known cardiac conditions or concerns throughout life. If the deceased is an adult, it may be helpful to gain childhood information from the parent of the deceased. Finally, obtain details around the circumstances of the death event. How was the victim feeling that day? Were there any complaints or symptoms expressed? Were there any unusual activities performed? Were there any unusual environmental conditions that could have led to the death event (i.e., driving late at night, swimming, extreme sports, etc.)? Was the event witnessed? If so, are there details that can be provided? Given the emotional nature of these questions, it is critical to provide the family the appropriate amount of time to gather thoughts, express their feelings, and calmly work through the process.

Next, we turn to family history and the development of a family pedigree. Information should be solicited from knowledgeable family members regarding siblings, parents, grandparents, and other relatives who may have suffered from similarly tragic circumstances. Of note, this may need to take place over several visits or taking the time to allow family members to call each other to sort out the medical history as you ask questions. It is not uncommon to be in an office visit while on the phone with a family member across the country who is answering questions about estranged relatives.

Frankly speaking, none of these important questions and clinical investigation can be accomplished in a 30-minute visit. The appropriate amount of time must be allocated and may require a spread over multiple visits and with multiple family members. The opportunity must not be taken lightly as discovering the nature of the event and what may have led to it will help provide a plan for further testing and evaluation of all first-degree relatives for inheritable conditions.

Diagnostic testing

An ECG and echocardiogram are reasonable tests to order on a first degree relative of a presumed victim of sudden unexplained cardiac death at a young age. The focus of the ECG is to review for electrical conditions that may suggest an arrhythmic related death, while the focus of the echocardiogram is to look for structural heart disease. If the deceased family member has a history of an ECG or echocardiogram previously performed, this would be beneficial for review. If physical activity was related to the circumstances of the death, it may be worth pursuing an exercise stress test. Other testing that a pediatric electrophysiologist may employ could include a medication challenge, Holter or other forms of ambulatory ECG monitoring, cardiac MRI, signal-averaged ECG, or diagnostic electrophysiology study depending on the suspected condition.

Genetic testing revealing a known mutation for a specified disease is becoming the standard for diagnosis. A coordinated effort between the local medical examiner and those investigating for sudden cardiac death can help ensure that genetic material is made available for testing. It is recommended to keep 5—10 mL of whole blood in EDTA containing tubes (purple top) that can be frozen. If blood is not available, cardiac or any body tissue can be used for genetic testing. Given that such requests are by definition unexpected, the wise cardiologist has preemptively educated the local emergency rooms, medical examiners and the like about this issue so that they have an actionable plan when dealing with a sudden unexplained death, particularly in the young. A positive genetic test in a deceased family member for a known mutation specific to a disease state can help provide the most appropriate testing for other family members to identify those at risk. However, genetic testing can also demonstrate variants of unknown significance. These are identified mutations that are not known to be disease-causing but may be consistent within a specified region of the genetic sequence that can contain known disease-causing mutations. These mutations should be reviewed with the help of a genetic counselor and pediatric cardiologist specializing in genetic arrhythmia or structural cardiac disease.

Action plan

The suspicion for cardiac-related sudden death is high for the patient in the scenario. A pediatric cardiology consultation should be performed with emphasis on history taking and a clear understanding of the potential conditions the deceased family member may have had before the event. Family history should be thoroughly reviewed and may require further conversation with family members outside the immediate family while documenting a family pedigree. All first-degree relatives of the decedent should be screened. An ECG and echocardiogram are usually an acceptable place to start for evaluation of cardiac disease, but further testing may be required depending on the suspected differential. Due to the time-sensitive nature of genetic testing, an early conversation should be held with the medical examiner or coroner to review the need for two 5—10 mL EDTA purple top lab tubes of blood that can be frozen for future genetic testing. Once the sample has been confirmed obtained, further discussions into the pros and cons of genetic testing can be held with the family, preferably with a genetic counselor, including its limitations and associated costs. In the scenario of no demonstrable diagnosis with genetic testing, DNA can be banked by various institutions for future testing should the need arise.

Suggested readings

Ackerman MJ, Priori SG, Willems S, et al. HRS/EHRA expert consensus statement on the state of genetic testing for the channelopathies and cardiomyopathies this document was developed as a partnership between the Heart Rhythm Society (HRS) and the European Heart Rhythm Association (EHRA). *Heart Rhythm*. 2011;8(8):1308—1339. https://doi.org/10.1016/j.hrthm.2011.05.020.

Lahrouchi N, Raju H, Lodder EM, et al. Utility of post-mortem genetic testing in cases of sudden arrhythmic death syndrome. *J Am Coll Cardiol*. 2017;69(17):2134—2145. https://doi.org/10.1016/j.jacc.2017.02.046.

Middleton O, Baxter S, Demo E, et al. National association of medical examiners position paper: retaining postmortem samples for genetic testing. *Acad Forensic Pathol*. 2013;3(2):191—194. https://doi.org/10.23907/2013.024.

7-year-old, asymptomatic, with ECG obtained for physical demonstrating WPW

13

Case

Hi thanks for taking my call. I'm a local psychiatrist and I obtained an ECG on this 7-year-old boy who I follow and was recently diagnosed with ADHD. The reading from the ECG machine says it is "abnormal" with a comment at the top saying "Evidence of Ventricular Preexcitation." The child has been asymptomatic and has never complained of any heart related concerns to my knowledge. I am wondering if it is OK to start him on ADHD medications or if I should have him see you?

What am I thinking?

My first reaction is to get a copy of this ECG sent to me for my direct review. If the ECG does show evidence of preexcitation then we are most likely dealing with a child with asymptomatic Wolff-Parkinson-White (WPW) syndrome. This brings up two issues; namely the issue of asymptomatic WPW and how best to manage that, and secondly, the safety of ADHD medications in someone with WPW. In this case, given the desire to start ADHD medications, I would recommend that the child be seen by a pediatric cardiologist or electrophysiologist to meet with the family and discuss the benefits and risks. We will also have an opportunity to discuss the management of WPW and what options we might have to pursue.

Tachycardias possible with WPW	QRS appearance
Atrioventricular reentrant, orthodromic (down AV node)	Narrow
Atrioventricular reentrant, antidromic (down accessory pathway)	Wide
Atrial fibrillation with rapid ventricular response (via accessory pathway)	Wide
AV nodal reentrant tachycardia (bystander pathway- not involved)	Narrow

Arrhythmias in Children. https://doi.org/10.1016/B978-0-323-77907-4.00013-5

History and physical

The first step for evaluating a child with a WPW pattern on ECG is to elicit any history of symptoms. Symptoms can include a feeling of tachycardia or heart racing as well as syncope. Depending on the age of the child, this can sometimes be difficult to elicit. Using colloquial descriptions such as "heart beating out of your chest," "fast beeping heart," and other terms may provide a better history from the patient. Requesting history from the parents about times in which the child complained about the heart or chest may also be helpful keeping in mind that complaints can often be nonspecific.

The estimated prevalence of WPW is approximately 1–3 per 1000 individuals. WPW pattern on ECG demonstrates a shortened PR interval with a widening of the QRS and lack of Q waves (see Figs. 13.1 and 13.2A). This is created by the presence of an accessory pathway that bypasses the typical atrioventricular node allowing for excitation of the ventricle before the normal conducting His-Purkinje system (i.e., ventricular preexcitation). Most accessory pathways can result in the risk of a reentrant form of SVT. This can be by conducting down the AV node and back up the pathway, termed orthodromic, which would result in a narrow complex tachycardia. This can also be by conduction down the pathway and up the AV node, termed

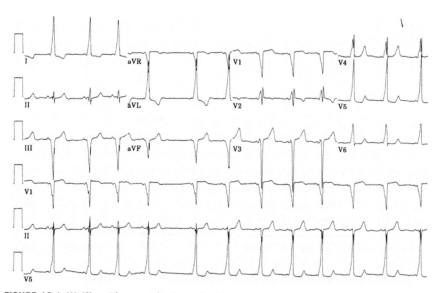

FIGURE 13.1 Wolff-parkinson-white (WPW) ECG.

Demonstration of ventricular preexcitation with a shortened PR segment and widening of QRS resulting in antegrade conduction through an accessory pathway fusing with conduction through the AV node. The ECG pattern of preexcitation will differ based on the location of the accessory pathway (contrast with Fig. 13.2).

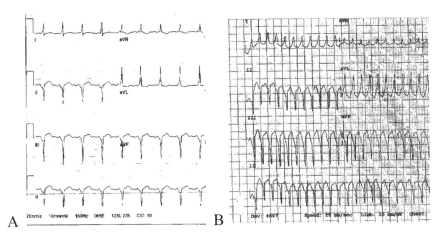

FIGURE 13.2 Wolff-parkinson-white (wpw) antidromic tachycardia.

(A) Limb lead ECG demonstration of WPW during sinus rhythm demonstrating fusion between accessory pathway and AV node conduction. (B) Tachycardia in the same patient demonstrating antidromic conduction in which antegrade conduction is exclusively through the accessory pathway and retrograde through the AV node. This results in a fully preexcited or wide complex tachycardia. This may be confused for ventricular tachycardia but note the same conduction pattern during sinus rhythm. Given the involvement of the AV node, this type of tachycardia will terminate with disruption of AV nodal conduction (i.e., adenosine).

antidromic, which would result in a wide complex tachycardia. This wide complex tachycardia may be confused for a ventricular tachycardia (see Fig. 13.2B).

The most concerning arrhythmia that a patient with WPW is at risk for is what is known as preexcited atrial fibrillation. Atrial fibrillation is very rare in children, but, for unclear reasons, occurs more frequently in patients with WPW. In the absence of an accessory pathway (in normal persons), the ventricular rate during atrial fibrillation tends to be slow because of the "protective" properties of the AV node that does not allow rapid conduction to the ventricle and thereby keeps the ventricular rate at a reasonable level. In patients with an accessory pathway, the ventricular rate becomes dependent on the refractory period of the accessory pathway. In patients with WPW and an accessory pathway capable of rapid conduction (due to a short refractory period), the patient may deteriorate into ventricular fibrillation (see Figs. 13.3 and 13.4). This arrhythmia is life-threatening and can result in sudden cardiac death but that is entirely dependent on the conduction properties of the accessory pathway. A rapidly conducting accessory pathway may be capable of transmitting an atrial fibrillation rate of 250–300 bpm to the ventricle, essentially resulting in ventricular fibrillation and sudden death.

Family history is usually reviewed for other members that may have had a history of WPW. It is extremely rare to have a family history of WPW and most WPW cases are sporadic. Family screening with ECG for WPW is not a recommendation when preexcitation is discovered in an individual. Physical examination is most often

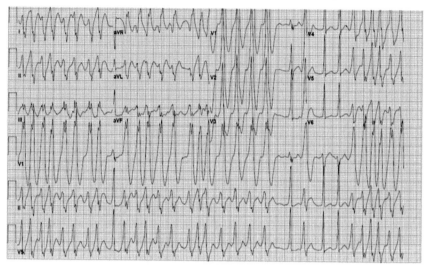

FIGURE 13.3 Atrial fibrillation in wolff-parkinson-white (WPW).

ECG demonstrates an irregular, chaotic, wide complex tachycardia occurring as a result of atrial fibrillation conducting rapidly to the ventricle via a WPW accessory pathway. Rapid ventricular response due to WPW can degenerate into ventricular fibrillation and result in sudden death. As the arrhythmia is atrial fibrillation and does not involve the AV node, disruption of AV nodal conduction (adenosine) will not terminate the arrhythmia. Immediate synchronized cardioversion is utilized to terminate the atrial fibrillation.

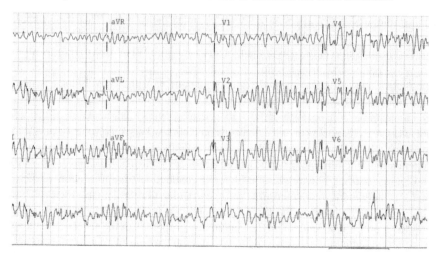

FIGURE 13.4 Ventricular fibrillation.

ECG demonstrates ventricular fibrillation. Patient was supported by cardiopulmonary bypass and ECG was obtained to determine the underlying rhythm. Gain was set to 20 mm/mV to better see waveforms as at standard gain (10 mm/mV) the signal was too small (i.e., "fine" ventricular fibrillation).

normal in WPW patients as the condition is associated with electrical changes. There is an association between WPW and Ebstein's anomaly as well as hypertrophic cardiomyopathy conditions (i.e., Danon's disease) that may manifest with physical examination findings.

Diagnostic testing

The electrocardiogram is the diagnostic test of choice for WPW and will often demonstrate the ventricular preexcitation pattern previously described. Again, computer interpretations will often miss the subtle changes of preexcitation emphasizing the need for trained interpretation by a medical professional. Age may also affect the presentation of the ECG as infants may demonstrate WPW but lose the preexcitation beyond a year of life in approximately 40% of cases.

An echocardiogram should be obtained on patients with WPW pattern to evaluate for structural heart disease and cardiac function. Ebstein's anomaly is the most common congenital heart disease associated with the WPW pattern though others have also been associated. Hypertrophic cardiomyopathy patients have also been demonstrated to have preexcitation. On rare occasions, ventricular preexcitation can result in a dyssynchronous contraction of the ventricle leading to a depressed ejection fraction over time. Finally, ensuring a structurally normal heart can help with the planning of further studies including EP study.

Action plan

For the patient described in the clinical scenario, a pediatric cardiologist evaluation should be obtained. An ECG and echocardiogram will likely be ordered and reviewed. In the case of the truly asymptomatic WPW patient, another testing may be considered to help risk stratify. Holter monitoring may provide evidence of intermittent changes in WPW pattern with loss of ventricular preexcitation. Exercise testing may also be performed to determine if at higher heart rates if ventricular preexcitation disappears suggesting poor antegrade properties of the pathway. The intermittent nature of ventricular preexcitation can be reassuring but does not exclude, with certainty, the possibility of arrhythmic arrest.

In many respects, the doctors and family are left with a risk-benefit decision in the patient with ADHD and asymptomatic WPW. It is known that stimulant medication can increase the resting heart rate by 1−2 bpm, which is felt to be not clinically relevant. The influence of this on the WPW population is not well studied. At present, the recommendation is that any patient with a known WPW pattern can be started on ADHD medications while monitoring for symptoms under the supervision of a pediatric cardiologist and their ordering physician. For most children, the benefit of ADHD medications on school performance, activities, and personal life far outweigh the risk associated with their usage. In a child with asymptomatic

WPW, the risk may be slightly higher but unlikely to alter the final decision. Regardless, asymptomatic WPW may provoke significant anxiety and concern among all participants due to the risk of sudden cardiac death. As a result, the Pediatric and Congenital Electrophysiology Society have published clinical guidelines for the management of the asymptomatic WPW patient and research continues to be performed to better define those at risk. Those patients 8 years and older who have persistent, WPW pattern conduction at maximal heart rates during an exercise stress test or Holter monitor during exercise, are recommended to undergo an invasive risk stratification procedure (intracardiac or transesophageal) to assess accessory pathway conduction properties (class IIA). The assessment of pathway conduction is performed by inducing atrial fibrillation and documenting the cycle length of the SPERRI or spontaneous preexcitation R-R interval. This is performed by measuring the shortest interval between two preexcited beats during an atrial fibrillation episode. An SPERRI of less than 250 ms (ventricular rate >240 bpm) is considered a high risk for sudden cardiac death. In the pediatric population, impact of catecholamines, suppression by sedation or anesthesia, and a nonactive state may influence the SPERRI and the interpretation. In the setting of an intracardiac EP study, identification of pathway location and inducibility of SVT can also be performed. Here again, weighing risk and benefit may suggest the pursuance of an ablation strategy to eliminate antegrade pathway conduction, thereby eliminating the risk for sudden cardiac death. While highly desirable, this must be weighed against the risks of ablation and damage to surrounding structures of the pathway that may include the AV node and/or coronary arteries. However, the elimination of pathway conduction *when safe* is the preferred and most often pursued strategy in the pediatric population.

Suggested reading

Pediatric and Congenital Electrophysiology Society (PACES), Heart Rhythm Society (HRS), American College of Cardiology Foundation (ACCF). PACES/HRS expert consensus statement on the management of the asymptomatic young patient with a Wolff-Parkinson-white (WPW, ventricular preexcitation) electrocardiographic pattern: developed in partnership between the Pediatric and Congenital Electrophysiology Society (PACES) and the Heart Rhythm Society (HRS). Endorsed by the governing bodies of PACES, HRS, the American College of Cardiology Foundation (ACCF), the American Heart Association (AHA), the American Academy of Pediatrics (AAP), and the Canadian Heart Rhythm Society (CHRS). *Heart Rhythm.* 2012;9(6):1006–1024. https://doi.org/10.1016/j.hrthm.2012.03.050.

Adolescent

15-year-old with intentional ingestion of grandparent's heart rhythm medication

---

Case

I'm calling from the ER and I have a 15-year-old female that has just been brought in by paramedics for a drug overdose. She is responsive to pain but non-communicative. This is her second suicide attempt according to the family. She lives with her grandparents and apparently they found her in her room surrounded by empty bottles of her grandfather's heart medication. I'm not sure what she has taken but her heart rate is only 40 bpm. Her blood pressure is low at 92/50 and she responds to pain and stimuli but she's non-communicative. I have poison control on the other line but given that there's heart medication involved, I reached out to you as well. Any idea what I should do from here?

What am I thinking?

This call is unfortunately becoming all too common. My initial thoughts are focused on how to support the child and calling poison control in the event of an intentional ingestion is absolutely the right first call. We should start with supportive care of the patient and make sure that she is stable while following instructions from poison control. The next thought is to gain some understanding of the type of medication taken and how much was taken. Given the low heart rate and blood pressure, my concern is that of a calcium channel blocker or β-blocker overdose.

Arrhythmias in Children. https://doi.org/10.1016/B978-0-323-77907-4.00014-7

ECG findings of antiarrhythmic drug overdose

Antiarrhythmic drug overdose	ECG findings
Digoxin	Scooping of ST segment
β-Blocker	Bradycardia, PR prolongation, AV block
Calcium channel blocker	Bradycardia, AV block, asystole
Sodium channel blocker	Widening QRS, ventricular arrhythmias
Potassium channel blocker	QT prolongation, AV block, Torsades de Pointes

History and physical

A focused history is often required in the aftermath of an intentional ingestion patient with an emphasis on what may have been ingested. The ingested medications may be prescribed for the individual who took the overdose but may also be medications used by other family members as described in the scenario. Trying to determine what pills were taken and how much of them will provide a concentrated approach to treatment. Past medical history to include medication history and other medical diagnoses may help with drug–drug interactions and systemic findings such as renal or hepatic impairment. As treatment is focused on supportive care, physical exam would be concentrated on demonstrating hemodynamic stability. Frequent recording of the vital signs including heart rate and blood pressure with attention to perfusion of the extremities via pulse and capillary refill should be the key. With ingestion of antiarrhythmic drugs, any evidence for shock is likely to be cardiac in origin.

Diagnostic testing

Laboratory workup should include a blood and urine toxicology screen for any other substances that may have been ingested. Standard labs such as arterial blood gas, lactate, chemistry panel to look for blood glucose, electrolyte changes, and evidence for other organ damage such as the liver and kidneys should be obtained. In the case of a suspected or known digoxin overdose, a serum digoxin level should be obtained. An ECG should be obtained to determine any significant rhythm disturbance such as varying degrees of AV block or changes to the QRS, T waves, and QT prolongation. Ingestion of a β-blocker or calcium channel blocker may present in cardiogenic shock and an echocardiogram should be ordered to evaluate the myocardial function. Additional labs and tests may be required per poison control/toxicology recommendations.

Action plan

A plan of action is largely driven by the known exposure and clinical presentation of the patient. Consultation with poison control centers and adherence to their recommendations is of utmost importance. Common in all scenarios is the required careful observation of rhythm and patient hemodynamic stability. In all intentional ingestion cases, once toxicity is under control and hemodynamic stability has returned without concern for arrhythmias, psychiatric assistance is required. Long-term cardiac care follow-up is not required. All ingestions are a cry for help and require intensive treatment by a trained mental health specialist. The following highlights generally acceptable actions for encountered cardiac drugs in intentional ingestions. However, a common consideration for almost all ingestions of medications that can cause severe myocardial depression is the use of mechanical cardiac support such as extracorporeal membrane oxygenation (ECMO) or a ventricular assist device. The details of such treatment are beyond the scope of this book, but faced with a major overdose ingestion, the decision to call for help from advanced practitioners should be made as early as possible.

Digoxin

Digoxin toxicity may manifest with nausea, vomiting, hyperkalemia, hypokalemia, bradycardia, and/or tachyarrhythmias. A digoxin level, while helpful, may not predict toxicity as patients may manifest differently to varying levels. The ECG changes are characteristic of a "scooping" of the ST segment. Patients suspected of an intentional overdose of digoxin may benefit from a dose of activated charcoal though this should be cleared by toxicology experts. Patients should be admitted for observation under cardiac monitoring as toxicity usually peaks 6 hours after the last dose. Supportive treatment of bradycardia may involve cardiac medications such as atropine, isoproterenol, and/or rarely require cardiac pacing. Correction of potassium abnormalities may be beneficial in minimizing the effects of digoxin toxicity. Hyperkalemia can be treated with insulin that drives potassium into cells. Hypokalemia can also occur in patients who have vomiting or diarrhea. Hypokalemia should be corrected as it exacerbates the cardiotoxic effects of digoxin. In the setting of severe hemodynamic compromise due to bradycardia or ventricular arrhythmias, administration of antidigoxin Fab may be recommended by toxicology experts. Antidigoxin Fab has a high binding affinity for digoxin and removes it from sodium-potassium-ATPase thereby reducing its cardiac toxicity.

β-blockers

Initial treatment of β-blocker ingestion is supportive. Fluid boluses may be required to manage hypotension. Toxicology may recommend a dose of activated charcoal. Severe clinical presentation is primary hypotension, bradycardia, and cardiac dysfunction resulting in cardiogenic shock. Treatment of cardiogenic shock should be performed in an intensive care unit under the supervision and instruction of a poison control center/toxicologist assisted by critical care and/or cardiology. An accepted treatment for cardiogenic shock due to β-blocker ingestion includes the use of high-dose insulin euglycemic therapy, epinephrine, and phosphodiesterase inhibitors such as milrinone. As some β-blockers can have sodium channel blocking activity (propranolol), other clinical manifestations can include changes to QRS morphology, arrhythmia, and seizure activity. Treatment for sodium channel blockers will be reviewed in a later section.

Calcium-channel blockers

The initial treatment of calcium-channel blocker ingestion is largely supportive. Determination of the type of calcium-channel blocker will be an important distinction for clinical presentation and treatment. Many calcium channel blockers have sustained or extended-release formulations that could result in delayed toxicity. Calcium channel blockers such as verapamil or diltiazem have both cardiotoxic and vasodilatory effects while dihydropyridine calcium channel blockers (such as amlodipine) mainly cause vasodilation. Primary treatment may require activated charcoal. Intravenous fluids may be used to manage hypotension. For severe cases of hypotension and/or cardiogenic shock, administration of high-dose insulin euglycemic therapy along with chronotropic medications may be necessary under intensive care. For dihydropyridine ingestions, vasopressor medications such as norepinephrine may need to be utilized. Calcium infusion may be considered under the direction of intensive care and cardiology.

Sodium channel blocker

Sodium channel blocker toxicity manifests clinically as nausea, vomiting, and seizures. ECG findings demonstrated widening of the QRS and development of ventricular arrhythmia. Medications such as flecainide are difficult to manage as they have a high oral bioavailability and slow rate of elimination. Treatment involves administration of high-dose hypertonic sodium bicarbonate that increases sodium levels and results in serum alkalinization thereby offsetting the cardiotoxic effects of the drug. Given the high rate of ventricular arrhythmias, treatment should be held in intensive care units under strict cardiac monitoring. In rare instances, hemodynamic support in the form of extracorporeal membrane oxygenation may be required.

Potassium channel blockers

Potassium channel blockers result in QT prolongation that can set up for ventricular arrhythmias such as Torsades de Pointes or heart block. Continuous cardiac monitoring for arrhythmia disturbances is the mainstay of management for suspected potassium channel blocker overdose. For medications such as amiodarone, acute toxicity is a rare phenomenon given the large volume of distribution but lends to longer-lasting effects and therefore patients should be monitored for days after an ingestion. Beyond rhythm manifestations, patients may experience hypotension, nausea, dizziness, and headache. As with other medications, primary treatment with activated charcoal may be indicated to reduce gastric absorption. Serum potassium and magnesium levels should be monitored and maintained to avoid cardiac arrhythmias. Temporary pacing may be required for those patients in heart block. For patients in Torsades de Pointes, management consists of immediate cardioversion, magnesium, and acceleration/overdrive of heart rate by isoproterenol or with pacing. Serial ECGs should be obtained until normalization of the rhythm and QTc interval have occurred.

Suggested readings

Campbell KB, Mando JD, Gray AL, Robinson E. Management of dofetilide overdose in a patient with known cocaine abuse. *Pharmacotherapy.* 2007;27(3):459–463. https://doi.org/10.1592/phco.27.3.459.

Graudins A, Lee HM, Druda D. Calcium channel antagonist and beta-blocker overdose: antidotes and adjunct therapies. *Br J Clin Pharmacol.* 2016;81(3):453–461. https://doi.org/10.1111/bcp.12763.

Roberts DM, Gallapatthy G, Dunuwille A, Chan BS. Pharmacological treatment of cardiac glycoside poisoning. *Br J Clin Pharmacol.* 2016;81(3):488–495. https://doi.org/10.1111/bcp.12814.

Vu NM, Hill TE, Summers MR, Vranian MN, Faulx MD. Management of life-threatening flecainide overdose: a case report and review of the literature. *Heart Rhythm Case Rep.* 2015;2(3):228–231. https://doi.org/10.1016/j.hrcr.2015.12.013.

16-Year-old with premature ventricular contractions noted during athletic participation physical

---

Case

Thanks for taking my call. I have this 16-year old adolescent male that I have been following for years who now presents for his athletic participation physical. As I am listening to his heart I am noting some skipped beats at rest. I don't recall ever hearing this before and I have nothing documented in his chart. He is completely asymptomatic and wants to play basketball this year and is trying out for the varsity team in a few weeks. He has been practicing regularly and has not had any symptoms. I think he should be fine but I'm a little nervous about clearing him with these extra beats. My plan is to send him for an ECG but I'm wondering if you would suggest anything else?

What am I thinking?

It would be good to characterize the type of extra beats or irregular rhythm that the doctor has noted and so an ECG is a good start. An irregular rhythm in a teen is usually the result of either prominent sinus arrhythmia, or else frequent ectopic beats more commonly due to premature ventricular contractions (PVC) and less commonly, premature atrial contractions (PAC). The question is then to determine if these are benign or the sign of something more malignant. Sinus arrhythmia refers to the prominent irregularity of sinus beats often seen in the young and related to the respiratory cycle. It is an entirely normal phenomenon and is diagnosed by a rhythm strip or ECG monitor showing that the beats are sinus in origin (similar looking p waves) but with a significant irregularity that waxes and wanes on the recording (see Fig. 8.1). Since it is a normal finding, all that is needed is reassurance. PACs that occur singly are not uncommon. Being frequent enough to be noticeable to a listening nurse or doctor is, however, surprisingly rare. They are generally benign and do not need further evaluation or management (see Fig. 2.2). PVCs are the most common cause of an obviously recognizable irregular heart rhythm in teenagers.

Differential diagnosis

Likely

Premature ventricular contractions
Normal sinus arrhythmia

Possible

Premature atrial contractions
Premature junctional beats
"Echo" beat from reentry

Rare

Intermittent AV block
Atrial fibrillation

A thorough history and physical can often find clues to provide a better context for these types of arrhythmias. Additional testing may be helpful including long-term monitoring and ruling out of structural heart disease by an echocardiogram. In most cases, premature ventricular contractions are benign in a healthy young person but obtaining some additional evidence to support that contention is necessary.

History and physical

Often in the case of an adolescent patient with premature ventricular contractions, the history and physical are entirely normal. History should be focused on any history of palpitations or syncope, particularly with activity. Family history should be thoroughly obtained to help guide toward a potential diagnosis of genetic arrhythmia syndrome. A review of the patient's dietary habits may be helpful, particularly the use of caffeinated beverages or energy drinks as these may lead to more ectopic beats. A review of medications is also important, particularly those that may result in electrolyte shifts (e.g., diuretics). Finally, the use of illicit drugs (steroids, cocaine, stimulants, etc.) may result in cardiac stress that could present with ectopic beats.

Physical examination is focused on cardiac findings to suggest cardiac disease. Auscultation of murmur may suggest structural heart disease though typically, the cardiac examination is normal with the exception of the ectopic beat upon auscultation. Changing the position of the patient from supine, to standing, to squatting may help elicit ectopic beats. Most often, the ectopic beats are noted while at rest. A reassuring sign is the suppression of ectopic beats with an increase in heart rate. Asking the patient to perform a physical activity such as jogging in place or jumping jacks in the office and then auscultating the heart again may show that the ectopic beats have gone away.

Diagnostic testing

Depending on the frequency of the ectopic beats, an ECG will be most helpful to identify the type and potential origin of the ectopic beat. PVCs have a distinct morphology suggesting the location of origin. On occasion, these PVCs may have more than one morphology and can be clearly delineated by changes in all of the ECG leads. Usually, a rhythm strip is required to capture enough of the PVCs that provides a comparison.

A 24-h Holter monitor is a good test to determine the frequency of the PVCs that can be helpful to determine additional steps required. Additionally, having the patient perform exercise during the Holter monitor provides the treating physician with a surrogate exercise stress test to demonstrate if PVCs increase with activity. Otherwise, a more traditional exercise stress test can be performed. For those patients who are symptomatic with their PVCs, it is recommended to keep a symptom diary with the Holter or use a cardiac event monitor to capture a single lead or multi-lead recording.

Blood chemistry to evaluate for electrolyte changes that may induce the PVCs is also recommended but is generally normal. In the setting of newly diagnosed PVCs, it is not unusual for an echocardiogram to be performed to evaluate for potential structural heart disease but also to evaluate for cardiac function. However, an echocardiogram is not always needed. A normal cardiac physical examination and normal appearance to the non-PVC sinus beats may be sufficient in many patients and echocardiography in such patients is of low yield. The real importance of echocardiography is in patients with a high (usually 20% or greater) PVC burden. PVC burden refers to the percentage of total beats that are due to PVCs. This number can be derived by Holter monitoring. Patients with a high burden may go on to develop ventricular dysfunction that is labeled as PVC-induced cardiomyopathy.

If history and physical are pointing to more concerning structural disease, a cardiac MRI may be helpful to evaluate for a scar related to hypertrophic cardiomyopathy or arrhythmogenic right ventricular cardiomyopathy.

Action plan

All young athletes who are noted to have premature ventricular contractions should be evaluated by a pediatric cardiologist. In most cases, these forms of arrhythmia are considered benign and do not pose any threat to the patient or their physical activity. However, there are some occasions where ventricular beats noted during activity may be the first sign of cardiovascular disease. Patients should undergo an ECG and Holter monitor at minimum. An echocardiogram could be considered if physical examination or the non-PVC sinus beat morphology is abnormal or if the PVC burden on Holter is high.

Depending on the results of the initial workup, further workup may be required. The asymptomatic young athlete with a structurally normal heart, normal cardiac function, and negative family history is likely to have benign ventricular ectopy. Benign ectopy is further supported with monomorphic morphology and low frequency that suppresses at higher heart rates.

Yet another important finding that supports a diagnosis of benign PVC is a patient who satisfies the above criteria and also has a characteristic morphology of PVCs that suggests that they arise from the right or left ventricular outflow tract (see Fig. 15.1). The characteristic pattern is one of PVCs with a left bundle branch block type of morphology with positive waves in leads II, III, and aVF, which suggest a high cardiac origin.

It is not unusual for such patients with benign PVCs to have short runs of bigeminy (every alternate beat is a PVC), couplets, triplets, or short runs of nonsustained ventricular tachycardia (VT) that is defined as a ventricular rhythm that either lasts less than 30 s and/or does not cause hemodynamic collapse (see Fig. 15.2). However, despite the word VT raising fear in the minds of many physicians, these patients have a benign prognosis and do not need to be treated differently from those without VT.

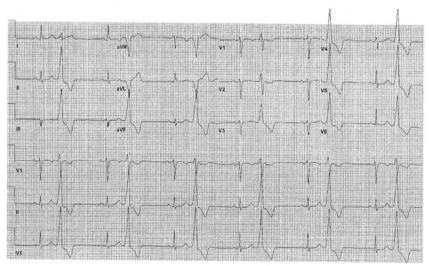

FIGURE 15.1 Outflow tract premature ventricular contraction.

ECG demonstrates a bigeminal pattern of premature ventricular contractions. The PVC beats appear upright in the inferior leads (II, III, aVF) demonstrating a superior to inferior conduction pattern. This suggests an origin in the ventricular outflow tracts.

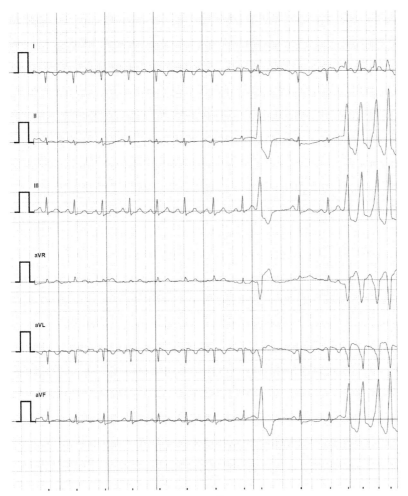

FIGURE 15.2 Nonsustained ventricular tachycardia.

Limb-lead ECG demonstration of PVC and subsequent monomorphic, nonsustained ventricular tachycardia at the end of the strip that lasted for four beats. Although not depicted, rhythm returned to sinus rhythm after this four-beat run.

Patients are educated about their arrhythmia and signs to watch for including recurrent or long-standing palpitations, near-syncope or syncope with exercise, and inability to keep up with peers. Caffeine and so-called "energy drinks" may exacerbate ectopic rhythms and appropriate hydration and nutrition are encouraged. These patients are allowed to participate in sports without restriction with annual follow-up to assess any changes in symptoms, ectopic frequency, or cardiac function.

13-Year-old with syncope while standing in line for lunch

16

Case

Hi, we have a 13-year old girl who was brought in by ambulance after she passed out today at school. She was standing in line at the cafeteria during lunchtime. The teacher reports that she fell to the ground while in line and woke up almost immediately. The teacher stated that she looked pale. She looks well now and the vitals are all stable. Should we be concerned? Should we do any testing?

What am I thinking?

This is a classic story for vasovagal syncope (VVS). However, I would want to make sure they are not missing something more dangerous. Vasovagal syncope (sometimes called by various other names like "simple" fainting, or the more scientific, "neurocardiogenic syncope") implies that the faint was due to loss of blood pressure maintaining reflexes with hypotension and fainting. It is extremely common and teenagers seem to be particularly more prone to such faints. There are typical scenarios where such fainting happens such as lined up in a crowded cafeteria and hungry (hypoglycemia as a factor). Studies have shown that 99% of faints in teenagers are due to VVS and only 1% have something concerning going on.

Common scenarios of vasovagal syncope in the child

Standing in line for lunch
Standing at religious services
Standing for performances (choir, marching band, parade)
Hair-combing or hair styling after hot shower
Postvomiting/diarrhea illness
Blood draws, injections, or other painful procedures
Sight of blood or other revolting sight to the victim
Postmicturition in males

Arrhythmias in Children. https://doi.org/10.1016/B978-0-323-77907-4.00016-0

History and physical

The most important aspect in evaluating someone who has fainted is the history. Attention should be paid to the detailed history of the event. Here, we have the history that the teenager was standing in the lunch line. VVS almost always happens while the person is either sitting or standing and almost never happens while the person is lying down. Another aspect to inquire is about dehydration and hunger. Was the patient ill in some way with diarrhea or vomiting? Has he or she not been drinking adequate liquids? Have they been not eating properly? A child who is late to school and runs out of the house not having had breakfast is much more likely to faint while standing in a cafeteria lunch line.

Other scenarios where fainting often occurs due to loss of blood pressure are while prolonged standing (parade ground, marching band, church), sudden standing, hypoglycemia, dehydration, during micturition in boys, during hairstyling or combing while standing in girls, after a sudden painful event (such as having blood drawn or an injection), or after seeing something scary or revolting (the sight of blood for example). Fainting is more common in hot weather or environments.

VVS is often, though not always, accompanied by a typical prodrome that consists of descriptions like tunnel vision, a headache or a heavy-headed feeling, nausea, feeling hot all over, feeling cold all over, and/or a numbness or tingling sensation in various parts of the body. Witnesses may describe the patient as pale or diaphoretic before the faint. Fainting during the act of physical exercise should be assumed to be a dangerous faint unless proven otherwise. Fainting minutes after completion of a physically challenging event is often VVS (see Chapter 17), but it is better to exercise caution and be more thorough in all exercise-related faints.

The loss of consciousness during VVS is typically brief. There may be stiffening of the body or, rarely, a shivering type movement. Eye rolling can happen. Rhythmic jerky movements are rare and should suggest a seizure as the cause. Incontinence of bowel or bladder is almost never present in VVS. Physical recovery after VVS is typically rapid and complete although some fatigue may persist for the remainder of the day.

An important question to ask in the history is to see if there has been any family member who has died in a sudden or unexplained manner. This may include specifically asking if anyone went to sleep and never woke up, if someone who knew swimming was found drowned, unusual and hard to explain car accidents (where the person may have passed out before the accident). The presence of such a history increases the likelihood that there may be an underlying hereditary condition (like hypertrophic cardiomyopathy or long QT syndrome) that is associated with sudden death. Long QT syndrome has a specific and peculiar association with death during swimming and also with passing out after a sudden, alarming noise.

Physical examination is normal in patients with VVS. Examination should focus on ruling out concerning findings for cardiac disease such as rhythm abnormalities or additional cardiac sounds such as murmurs, rubs, or gallops. Assessment of hydrational status may also be useful for further management.

Diagnostic testing

In most patients where the history is highly suggestive of VVS, the only test that helps is a standard ECG. The ECG can help identify cardiomyopathy, long QT, and Wolff Parkinson White (rare cause of sudden death). If the history is clear, physical exam unremarkable, and ECG is normal, a diagnosis of VVS can be made with confidence. It is particularly important to avoid wasteful tests like CT scan of the brain, EEG, and echocardiograms, as their yield is usually extremely low in the patient with classic presentation of VVS.

Patients with exercise-associated syncope should get an echocardiogram, mainly to look for cardiomyopathy (hypertrophic cardiomyopathy being the most common offender) and to look specifically at the origins and initial course of the coronary arteries. An anomalous left coronary artery coming off the right-facing sinus and winding its way with an intramural (inside the vessel wall) course is the most common congenital coronary anomaly associated with exercise-induced ventricular fibrillation and sudden death. Less frequently, one may detect an anomalous right coronary artery arising from the right sinus and then going to the left. While reduced cardiac function is easy to detect, identifying the coronary arteries reliably by echocardiogram needs experience and skill, which is not something that can be done by a quick point of care echocardiogram. If the echocardiogram is normal and there is still concern about the syncope, other tests to consider would be an exercise test (if the syncope was associated with exercise), or a Holter or longer ECG monitor to try and catch the ECG during an episode.

Action plan

Management of VVS basically consists of reassurance that it will improve as the child gets older and encouraging a diet higher in salt and increased water intake. Patients should be encouraged to drink at least 64 oz of noncaffeinated beverages per day and add a daily salty snack to their diet. Patients are advised that when their prodrome occurs and they feel "faint," they should immediately lay down with their legs up to help prevent injury and improve symptoms. In fact, one may say that VVS is nature's way of telling someone to lie down.

Most patients respond well to these simple measures. Those who fail this will usually need a specialist referral. Anxiety and emotional stress are commonly associated with fainting. Patients with an anxiety disorder can be complex to manage and would not be amenable to standard VVS treatment. Specialist psychology or psychiatry referral should be strongly considered.

The 1% of patients who have something else more malignant are either those with a seizure disorder mistakenly diagnosed as a faint, or else cardiac conditions that put them at risk for cardiac arrest and sudden death. Such cardiac conditions include cardiomyopathies, channelopathies like long QT syndrome, or else abnormal coronary arteries (see Chapter 18). The common factor in all is the etiology of lethal ventricular arrhythmias. Therefore, the "faint" may be a warning that something more serious could happen.

14-Year-old cross country runner presents with syncope during a race

17

Case

Hi, I'm calling from the ER and sorry to bother you on a weekend. I have this 14-year old female who has been previously healthy and passed out while she was running in her first high-school cross-country race this morning. When she came in by paramedics who were at the race, she looked a bit pale and sweaty but she did just run the race. I gave her some fluids and she seems to be feeling better. Her vital signs are stable but her heart rate was a bit up at 95 bpm when she first came in. I'm thinking about sending her home after her fluids are up but I'm sure you heard about that young kid in the town over that died while running track a few months ago. They say it was related to his heart so I just wanted to make sure I checked with you before sending her home. Anything else I should do?

What am I thinking?

I am continually amazed by what young people are capable of when they put they make up their minds and push their bodies beyond natural limits. Of all the physical activities that we encounter in young people, cross country running seems to result in frequent episodes of syncope during competitive meets. The concept of syncope during physical activity is concerning and rightfully so as a harbinger of serious cardiac disease. However, history taking often finds that the athlete syncope patient may not be passing out in midactivity, but often postactivity when the dedicated and driven young-person crosses that finish line. In the eternal struggle of mind over the body, the mind often wins the battle but the body eventually and inevitably wins the war.

Arrhythmias in Children. https://doi.org/10.1016/B978-0-323-77907-4.00017-2

Differential diagnosis
Likely
Neurocardiogenic or vasovagal syncope - Vasodepressor, cardioinhibitory or mixed type
Possible
Heatstroke Illicit drug use
Rare
Hypertrophic cardiomyopathy Anomalous coronary artery Wolff-Parkinson-White Catecholaminergic polymorphic ventricular tachycardia Arrhythmogenic right (or left) ventricular dysplasia Long QT syndrome Brugada syndrome

History and physical

As has been mentioned previously in this book, a thorough and detailed history is paramount to the clinical evaluation of patients suffering syncope. In many ways, it can be compared to a crime scene investigation in which details are gathered from all eyewitnesses to put together a reenactment of the event in question. Given the importance of such history-taking, it is imperative that the appropriate time be taken (and allotted) for such an evaluation. Part of the evaluation often involves asking questions repeatedly to get a clear answer as patients and parents will often report the main event skipping over multiple details that can help tease out the differential diagnosis.

First, an understanding of the circumstances of the event can be helpful. Was this a typical day or a special event (i.e., sports practice, race day, etc.)? Where was everyone located and who witnessed the event? What was the environmental climate during the event (i.e., hot day outside vs. indoors)? Excessive heat combined with strenuous physical activity can lead to heatstroke. What was the general feeling of the patient before the event: history of previous illness? Appropriate nutrition and hydration that day and days prior? Overall feeling of health?

A critical question to ask is to enquire when the event took place. Did this occur while participating in physical activity or was it afterward? In the case of a runner, was it during the actual run or minutes afterward in recovery? It is not uncommon for complaints of "syncope with exercise" to reach the pediatric cardiologist only to determine through a more detailed history that the event occurred after the race while drinking water. It is also not uncommon to hear stories of coaches or relatives encouraging young athletes to keep walking despite the feeling of dizziness and lightheadedness that eventually results in collapse.

Next, focus on the details of the event. What was the patient feeling and how were they acting according to eyewitnesses, minutes to seconds before the event? Those who experience a vagal-related syncope often experience symptoms of light-headedness, dizziness, and/or tunnel-vision without mention of unusual heartbeats or chest pain. How did the patient collapse: were they able to put their hands out to "catch" their fall or did they collapse without doing so, leading to injuries? Patients who were able to catch themselves as they fell usually have scratches and bruises on their extremities. How did the patient look when they were passed out? Usually, young people who have undergone a neurocardiogenic event during physical activity appear quite pale.

Next, focus on recovery. How long after the initial event did it take for the patient to regain consciousness? Was there a true loss of consciousness or loss of vision/hearing? Did anyone feel for a pulse or initiate resuscitative efforts? In the case of the neurocardiogenic athlete, the loss of consciousness is quite brief with the almost immediate regaining of consciousness once blood flow has been restored to the brain—usually seconds after the head falls to the ground. Ask the young athlete how they felt for the rest of the day? The neurocardiogenic syncope victim is often quite exhausted from their "fight or flight" adrenaline response.

Family history is also important to rule out a genetically inherited disease. Questions should include any family member that suffered an unexplained death such as an unexplained car accident or drowning. Questions should be asked about family members with unexplained seizures or deaths while playing sports-either in practice or in game. Ask about deaths presumed to be due to heart attack before the age of 50 years, which may be in fact a sign of arrhythmic death.

In the adolescent, a proper social history can be lifesaving. This should involve interviewing the adolescent with parents or family out of the room and a chaperone present. Always ensure confidentiality with the patient making sure to let them know that the only event in which confidentiality may be broken is if you felt their life was in danger. Ask politely for their honesty and reassure that the questions asked are related to their health and for no additional purposes. Discuss home life, school life, and relationships. Review medication use, both prescribed and not prescribed as well as drugs of abuse. Victims of physical or sexual abuse may present with feigned syncope as a way of seeking help. Take the opportunity to ask about the potential for harm to themselves or others and ensure their feeling of safety at home. Ask if there is anything else the patient would like to share or ask while their family is out of the room. Finally, thank the adolescent for their honesty and express that they can always reach out if they have additional concerns.

Physical examination is often normal without evidence of cardiac disease manifesting as a pathologic murmur or rhythm change on auscultation. In the patient with a recent neurocardiogenic event (within hours), the patient may appear pale and fatigued. Abnormal body temperature is concerning for heatstroke. There may be bruises or scratches on the hands, forearms, or knees secondary to an attempt to catch themselves while falling.

Diagnostic testing

With a benign medical history and a story consistent with VVS or neurocardiogenic syncope, there are no specific tests that would be required except possibly an electrocardiogram. Often an electrocardiogram is ordered to rule out any obvious potential arrhythmic conditions. Patients are often seen in emergency rooms or urgent cares and it is not unusual to see an elevated specific gravity on urinalysis suggesting dehydration. There may be some slight electrolyte changes on serum chemistry panel as well.

Action plan

With the appropriate medical history details and normal physical, most patients who suffer syncope around the time of exercise and not during exercise are likely experiencing a form of neurocardiogenic syncope. If an ECG is performed it is most likely to present as normal. The primary method of treatment for neurocardiogenic syncope is to encourage hydration and intake of salt. The daily recommended amount of noncaffeinated beverages is 64 oz per day at baseline. With the addition of physical activities and loss by perspiration, this could mean additional ounces of fluid. This often requires a conscious effort to drink this amount of fluid. Urine should appear clear or straw colored but never dark yellow. Adding salt to the diet in the form of pickles, pretzels, or table salt to food will help. For those who tolerate it, salt tablets can be taken to help supplement and can be helpful for athletic competition. Although various pharmacological agents have been described (e.g., midodrine, fludrocortisone), water and salt alone are often enough to treat neurocardiogenic syncope. Exercise has also been shown to be helpful for these patients. Patients may return to activity and are encouraged to maintain adequate nutrition and hydration. Other possible factors that promote neurocardiogenic syncope are hypoglycemia (enquire if they missed a meal and were very hungry when they passed out), lack of sleep, concurrent illness (especially with fever or vomiting), and significant physical pain (abdominal colic, menstrual cramps, migraines, etc). For more difficult or recurrent cases, a pediatric cardiology evaluation may be indicated.

16-year-old athlete who has syncope during athletic competition

18

Case

I'm calling from the ER with a 16-year old male who was playing in a soccer tournament today and suddenly collapsed on the field. They say that just before he fell he was acting strange, a bit disoriented, and very unsteady on his feet. He was running the opposite direction of the ball and then he fell, face-first into the ground and has a pretty bad contusion to his forehead and may have broken his nose. An onlooker present at the game was a nurse and went to check on him when he wasn't getting up. She says that she may have felt a pulse but he really wasn't sure. She decided to start chest compressions and told people to call 9-1-1. After approximately 30 seconds of chest compressions the boy started to wake up and amazingly, wanted to get back in and play after paramedics had checked him out! He feels fine now except for his injuries to his face. I'm thinking that maybe he was just dehydrated but the "no pulse" thing kind of freaks me out. I'll get an ECG on him now but wondering if he needs to see you before playing again?

What am I thinking?

I need to see this young man and his family before he is cleared for sports again. Any discussion of pulselessness requires further evaluation involving history, family history, full physical examination, and a battery of tests to ensure current and future cardiac functioning. There are a number of conditions that can present in this similar circumstance and the answer may be found through cardiac and genetic testing for inherited cardiac arrhythmia syndromes. The scenario presented is that of an aborted sudden cardiac arrest until proven otherwise. Taking a logical and comprehensive approach to the evaluation will be key in determining the risk of a repeat event.

Differential diagnosis

Likely until excluded

Hypertrophic cardiomyopathy
Anomalous coronary artery
Wolff-Parkinson-White syndrome
Aortic stenosis
Myocarditis
Long QT syndrome
Catecholaminergic polymorphic ventricular tachycardia
Arrhythmogenic right (or left) ventricular cardiomyopathy
Brugada syndrome

Possible

Neurocardiogenic or vasovagal syncope
- Vasodepressor, cardioinhibitory, or mixed type

Heatstroke
Illicit drug use or prescription medication with side effect

Rare

Idiopathic ventricular fibrillation
Short QT syndrome
Early repolarization

History and physical

As was described in the previous chapter, the history taking is critical to an investigation of a syncopal patient. A meticulous and detailed history (e.g., "crime scene investigation") will lead to proper investigation and successful diagnosis. Such investigations take time and a significant amount of effort and should be conducted with the help of a pediatric cardiologist and/or electrophysiologist in cases such as the one described. Reaching out to eyewitnesses, first-responders, relatives often moves beyond the office visit and requires coordination. This chapter will focus on questions and answers that may lead the healthcare professional toward a structural or arrhythmic cardiac diagnosis.

Start with a history leading up to the event. On some occasions, victims of an aborted sudden cardiac arrest may have had a similar presentation earlier in their lives. Asking if the patient has ever suffered syncopal episodes in the past may lead to such discoveries. When asking about the minutes before the event, it is not uncommon for eyewitnesses to describe odd behavior. In patients experiencing arrhythmia, it is often reported that the patient was acting unusually before collapse; this is particularly true with sports participants (i.e., shooting an own goal, running the opposite way, standing in an awkward position). What does the patient recall about the fall: any prodrome of unusual heartbeats? Were any resuscitative measures used including the use of an automated external defibrillator? If so, were there any tracings from the defibrillator that could be obtained? Patients who have undergone a significant arrhythmia may not recall much of what happened before passing out and often awaken to discover that something had happened, but they feel ready to return to their previous activity. Those with arrhythmia who were unable to brace for a fall may result in significant facial injuries such as a broken nose, chipped teeth, and/or hematoma.

In a suspected aborted sudden cardiac arrest, the family history is critical to guiding toward a potential inherited diagnosis. Family history should focus on details of unexplained deaths in the family, unexplained drownings, unexplained seizures, and unexplained car accidents. Deaths related to physical activity or members of the family who have died of "heart conditions" before the age of 50 years. Specific conditions should be listed and asked for but the use of colloquial terms is encouraged for clear understanding (i.e., enlarged or thickened heart). Questions should also touch on possible aborted sudden cardiac arrest that usually manifests as syncope in specific situations. For example, asking about family members that pass out with loud noises (long QT syndrome) or with excitement such as roller coasters or being startled/surprised (catecholaminergic polymorphic ventricular tachycardia). Follow-up with relatives may be required for deaths in the family that may be unclear. The healthcare provider should be prepared to make additional phone calls that may involve difficult conversations with estranged family members.

The past medical history should investigate previous illness or syncopal episodes as well as recently taken medications. Genetic arrhythmia syndromes such as Long QT syndrome may be exacerbated by the use of prescribed or over the counter medications. Social history in the athlete should include determining the use of over the counter energy agents, performance-enhancing drugs, or illicit drug use.

Physical exam is focused on stigmata of cardiac disease that may manifest as unusual rhythm upon auscultation or a pathologic murmur. Generally, the physical examination is normal in patients with a condition that can lead to cardiac arrest making the history and additional testing so critical to diagnosis.

Diagnostic testing

A patient with this type of presentation will undergo a gamut of tests given the risk associated with aborted sudden cardiac arrest. In such cases, it is likely wise to admit the patient under cardiac monitoring for observation. Initial blood work should include cardiac enzymes (e.g., troponin I). Blood gas, chemistry panel, complete blood count, lactate, and toxicology screen should all be ordered to assess possible etiologies for the arrest and evaluation for end-organ damage. An ECG should be obtained to evaluate for a number of arrhythmic-related disease such as Wolff-Parkinson-White syndrome, Long QT syndrome, Brugada syndrome, or even myocarditis. It is recommended that serial ECGs be obtained given that some conditions may present with intermittently normal ECGs. An echocardiogram should be ordered to evaluate for structural heart disease including evaluation for anomalous origin or course of coronary arteries. An exercise stress test can act as a provocation test for arrhythmias in patients with catecholaminergic polymorphic ventricular tachycardia (see Fig. 18.1). Further testing may be required to elucidate the clinical, genetic, and anatomic factors that may have contributed to the cardiac arrest.

Cardiac MRI with delayed enhancement could help identify areas of scar for hypertrophic cardiomyopathy or fatty infiltrate for arrhythmogenic right ventricular cardiomyopathy. In some instances, cardiac CT or cardiac catheterization may help better characterize the origins and course of the coronary arteries. Consideration for electrophysiology study may also be considered. Drug challenges may also provoke cellular changes that can manifest as changes in ECG tracings and can be diagnostic in conditions such as Brugada syndrome or Long QT syndrome. For example, administration of procainamide can elicit the ST segment changes seen in Brugada patients (see Fig. 18.2). Administration of low-dose epinephrine has been demonstrated to result in prolongation of the QT interval in patients with Long QT syndrome, type 1.

Finally, genetic testing can be helpful in the aborted cardiac arrest patient and many companies offer genetic panels to screen for several mutations linked with

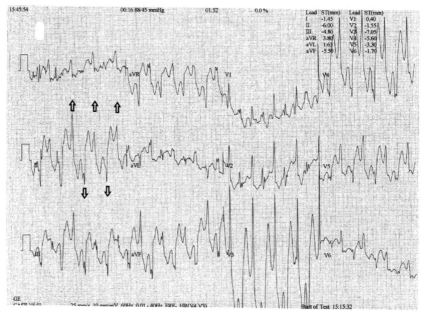

FIGURE 18.1 Bidirectional ventricular tachycardia.

ECG from an exercise stress test demonstrating a wide complex tachycardia that propagates in opposite directions (open arrows). This patient had a history of syncopal episodes with physical activity. The finding of bidirectional ventricular tachycardia was pathognomonic for catecholaminergic polymorphic ventricular tachycardia or CPVT.

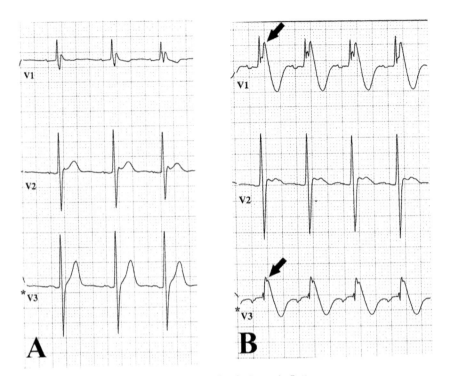

FIGURE 18.2 Procainamide challenge resulting in Brugada Pattern.

(A) Baseline ECG pattern of the anterior precordial leads V1, V2, and *V3, which was placed one intercostal space above the V2 position otherwise known as a V2B or Brugada position. (B) Procainamide was infused at 20 mcg/kg/min, which demonstrated a change in the leads with ST segment elevation (arrows) and pronounced T wave inversions suggestive of Brugada Syndrome. The patient had a febrile syncopal episode after being hospitalized for influenza and demonstrated ventricular arrhythmia on hospital monitoring provoking this drug challenge for diagnosis.

sudden cardiac death. While extremely helpful when diagnostic, at the time of this writing, gene panel testing may commonly be unclear. This is because many patients show variants of unknown significance or no known mutations associated with diseases known to be associated with sudden death.

Action plan

The presentation is concerning for sudden cardiac arrest and must involve consultation with a pediatric cardiologist and/or electrophysiologist. The patient should be admitted for observation under cardiac monitoring. A thorough history and physical examination should be performed followed by bloodwork, ECG, and echocardiogram to start. Further testing will be determined as evidence leads the practitioner down a path of diagnosis. If a diagnosis can be made and is found to be genetic in inheritance, this could lead to further testing of family members who may be affected. In the meantime, it is recommended that the patient be restricted from physical activity till such time that a clearer understanding of the risks and benefits of continued participation can be discussed with both the patient and family.

Suggested reading

Ackerman M, Atkins DL, Triedman JK. Sudden cardiac death in the young. *Circulation.* 2016;133(10):1006−1026. https://doi.org/10.1161/CIRCULATIONAHA.115.020254.

Maron BJ, Zipes DP, Kovacs RJ, American Heart Association Electrocardiography and Arrhythmias Committee of Council on Clinical Cardiology, Council on Cardiovascular Disease in Young, Council on Cardiovascular and Stroke Nursing, Council on Functional Genomics and Translational Biology, and American College of Cardiology. Eligibility and disqualification recommendations for competitive athletes with cardiovascular abnormalities: preamble, principles, and general considerations: a Scientific Statement from the American Heart Association and American College of Cardiology. *Circulation.* 2015; 132(22):e256−e261. https://doi.org/10.1161/CIR.0000000000000236.

17-year-old presents to emergency room with "irregularly irregular" rhythm

Case

Hello, I'm calling from the ER at the adult hospital across the street. I have a 17-year old male who came in for palpitations. He says that he first noted them two days ago when he was hanging out with his friends. They were playing basketball and he says he felt fine at that time but went to cool off with a drink at the local convenience store. I asked about energy drinks, but he says he just had one of those cold slush drinks. Soon after that he felt his heart beating funny. He went to bed that night and when he woke up he still had the same feeling but less pronounced. He's had school for the past few days so it wasn't bothersome enough to skip school but today he says that he's feeling more tired and has less energy than usual so his father brought him into the ER. When I auscultate, I hear an irregularly, irregular rhythm so I got an ECG. The ECG says that he is in atrial fibrillation! I tend to see a lot of this in our ER and it sure does look and sound like A-fib; but in a 17-year old? Should I start him on a diltiazem drip? Do I need to put him on anticoagulation?

What am I thinking?

I need to see this electrocardiogram. Atrial fibrillation is rare in the pediatric population but is possible. There may be other rhythms that could be mistakenly interpreted by the computer reading as atrial fibrillation. However, the presentation does sound characteristic of atrial fibrillation in a young adult. Given the unusual nature of this presentation, there are a number of assessments that will need to occur including history, family history, physical examination, echocardiogram, assessment of embolic risk, and ultimately decision regarding short and long-term management. In most cases, a cardioversion of the rhythm is indicated with follow-up for recurrences.

Arrhythmias in Children. https://doi.org/10.1016/B978-0-323-77907-4.00019-6

Causes of atrial fibrillation in the pediatric/adolescent population
Likely
Underlying congenital heart disease
SVT that degenerates into atrial fibrillation
Possible
Caffeine (energy drinks)
Cold medications (ephedrine)
Illicit drug use
Vagal mediated (cold drinks)
Rare
Thyrotoxicosis
Paroxysmal atrial fibrillation
Genetic arrhythmia syndrome

History and physical

Given the rarity of atrial fibrillation in the pediatric and adolescent population, the discovery of underlying substrates to set up this arrhythmia is often the primary focus for history taking. The past medical history should determine if the patient has a history of cardiac disease, either structural or electrophysiologic. For some clues, it is recommended to start with the history of present illness with specific importance as to the timing of the arrhythmia initiation as this can influence management. Additional information around surrounding environmental circumstances such as physical activity, medications, or food ingestions can be helpful. Patients have been known to present with atrial fibrillation after ingesting cold drinks such as slushies or ice cream shakes that have resulted in atrial fibrillation due to a vagal mediated response. Caffeinated beverages, stimulants such as ephedrine, or illicit drug use can induce ectopic beats that could be a set up for atrial fibrillation in the young patient. The determination of how often these types of arrhythmia symptoms are felt and with what frequency can be helpful to assess recurrence. Documentation of symptomatology will also be helpful to determine the need for ongoing monitoring. In most young people, the most common symptom is a feeling of palpitations and is often noted primarily at rest. Other associated symptomatology such as weight loss, feelings of anxiety, psychosis, and/or tremor may indicate a thyrotoxicosis. Neurologic symptoms such as weakness to one side, vision changes, dropping eyelids or lips, or speech disturbances would be highly concerning for cerebrovascular incidents (e.g., stroke, transient ischemic attack) and should be managed urgently. A family history of atrial fibrillation, particularly at a young age, may be indicative of a genetic arrhythmia syndrome.

Physical examination is usually normal in these patients, with the exception of those with underlying congenital heart disease. Atrial fibrillation may be the result of underlying conditions that serve as risk factors. These can include valvular heart disease, obesity, obstructive sleep apnea, systemic hypertension, diabetes mellitus type 2, and previous arrhythmias. As the young population becomes more obese and starts to develop disease states that are generally seen in adult populations, it is possible that atrial fibrillation will increase in the young. Cardiac auscultation should reveal the classically described "irregularly, irregular" rhythm portraying the chaotic activity of atrial fibrillation.

Diagnostic testing

An ECG is the best test to order for diagnosis of atrial fibrillation. This often demonstrates an undulating baseline that has an irregular pattern due to multiple p waves (see Fig. 19.1). ECGs should be interpreted by a pediatric cardiologist or ideally, an electrophysiologist. As atrial fibrillation is common in the adult population, ECG systems have an increased sensitivity to call irregular rhythms as atrial fibrillation. This can be a confounding factor in pediatric patients presenting with normal sinus arrhythmia who are erroneously labeled by the computer as having atrial fibrillation.

Action plan

Once the diagnosis of atrial fibrillation is established, the timing of the arrhythmia initiation should be elicited. Some patients may recollect the exact time they started feeling the palpitations that can be a helpful piece of history. As the arrhythmia creates a chaotic rhythm in the atria resulting in a lack of blood circulation, there

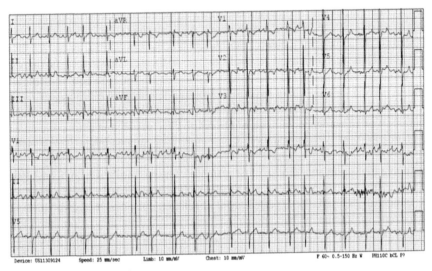

FIGURE 19.1 Atrial fibrillation.

ECG demonstrating chaotic atrial rhythm with varying ventricular conduction resulting in an irregular rhythm consistent with atrial fibrillation.

is an increased setup for thrombus formation. As a result, it is recommended to obtain imaging in a person who has had atrial fibrillation for greater than 48 h to evaluate for thrombus formation. A transesophageal echocardiogram is the preferred method of imaging due to the need for excellent imaging of the left atrial appendage that is most often the source of thrombus. In adults, patients may be started on therapeutic anticoagulation for a minimum of 3 weeks obviating the need for a transesophageal echocardiogram. In the adolescent experience, this is less likely to be the choice due to compliance concerns and the need for therapeutic monitoring. For those patients who present with atrial fibrillation for less than 48 h, a dose of heparin may be given before cardioversion, which is generally done as soon as feasible based on the availability of support staff and when it is safe to do so.

Cardioversion is performed utilizing the inpatient cardioverter/defibrillator under deep conscious sedation or anesthesia. The device should be synchronized to the QRS or "synched." It is recommended that patches be applied to the patient and energy selected to 0.5—1 J/kg of body weight. Failure to synchronize to the QRS may result in delivery of energy during a vulnerable period leading to ventricular fibrillation. Should this occur, immediate defibrillation (nonsynchronized) at 2—4 J/kg of body weight should be performed. In some patients, atrial fibrillation may be so long-standing that it requires multiple energy deliveries with escalating doses. Sometimes this requires repositioning of patches such as an anterior-posterior position rather than an anterior-left lateral position.

Once the patient has been successfully converted to sinus rhythm, the patient is monitored for recurrence before discharge. Recurrence is generally rare in the adolescent patient. When recurrence does occur, other considerations including the possibility of an additional arrhythmia substrate must be accounted. This can be seen in patients with accessory pathway-mediated atrioventricular reentrant tachycardia that eventually degenerates into an atrial fibrillation. Elimination of the underlying substrate for the arrhythmia may eliminate the cause of the atrial fibrillation. In adolescent patients with recurrent atrial fibrillation, an electrophysiology study is recommended to evaluate for additional substrates that may be amenable to ablation. Unlike in adults, pulmonary vein isolation is kept as a back-up option and used only in patients who fail less aggressive therapies.

Finally, a few words about anticoagulation and risk of stroke. The young adolescent is not often burdened with the additional risk factors seen in adult patients who are burdened with atrial fibrillation. Commonly used anticoagulant scores such as CHADS2VASC2, used in adults, are not applicable in adolescents as they usually fall into a low-score area. For the first instance of atrial fibrillation, anticoagulation is not generally recommended. An antiplatelet regimen such as 81 mg of aspirin may be empirically started. For repeated atrial fibrillation episodes, those who have had neurologic symptoms, or have previously demonstrated thrombus formation there may be an indication for anticoagulation, but this is quite rare. In the patient with significant risk factors for thrombus formation, anticoagulation may be utilized with the choice of anticoagulant determined after discussion between the patient, the family, and a pediatric cardiologist.

Suggested reading

Gourraud JB, Khairy P, Abadir S, et al. Atrial fibrillation in young patients. *Expert Rev Cardiovasc Ther.* 2018;16(7):489−500. https://doi.org/10.1080/14779072.2018.1490644.

January CT, Wann LS, Calkins H, et al. 2019 AHA/ACC/HRS focused update of the 2014 AHA/ACC/HRS guideline for the management of patients with atrial fibrillation: a report of the American College of Cardiology/American Heart Association Task Force on Clinical Practice Guidelines and the Heart Rhythm Society in Collaboration with the Society of Thoracic Surgeons [published correction appears in Circulation. 2019 Aug 6;140(6):e285] *Circulation.* 2019;140(2):e125−e151. https://doi.org/10.1161/CIR.0000000000000665.

Special circumstances

Maternal fetal evaluation reveals fetus with abnormal rhythm

20

Case

Hi, I'm a new obstetrician in town and I am seeing a mother who is 20 weeks along in her pregnancy. She has been handling the pregnancy well without any issue and this is the second pregnancy for the mother with the first resulting in live birth so she is a G2P1. Anyway, the reason I am calling is because when I was performing her ultrasound I noted that the fetal heart rate was very irregular and occasionally would go very fast. To me it sounds like an arrhythmia and I am concerned that it will affect the pregnancy. Is there someone I should be coordinating with to help manage the fetus? I know in my fellowship we coordinated with adult cardiology but when I called the local adult cardiologist they put me in touch with you. Any advice?

What am I thinking?

This sounds like a clear-cut case of a fetal arrhythmia. The issue, however, is figuring out: what type of arrhythmia, how serious it is for the fetus's health and development, and how to manage it. Management of fetal arrhythmias should be considered a team effort that involves a combination of the treating obstetrician, a fetal cardiologist, a pediatric electrophysiologist, and/or adult electrophysiologist. Decisions on who should be involved also depend on the suspected treatment plan that may additionally involve a cardiac surgeon.

Fetal arrhythmias can be simplified to bradyarrhythmias and tachyarrhythmias. Identification of the rhythm most commonly involves the use of a fetal echocardiogram and mechanical contraction of the atria and ventricles on an M-mode tracing that provides a surrogate electrocardiogram. A Doppler pattern of inflow and outflow from the left ventricle may act as a surrogate electrocardiogram as well. Fetal magnetocardiography can also, rarely, be utilized but is offered in limited centers.

Fetal bradycardia can be secondary to the development of fetal heart block. A fetus can present with varying degrees of heart block including first-degree, second-degree Mobitz I, second-degree Mobitz II, and third-degree or complete heart block. Infants born with heart block are at increased risk of having mothers who carry anti-SSA and anti-SSB antibodies. However, the converse is not true (i.e., mothers with anti-SSA and anti-SSB antibodies are not at higher risk for infants with heart block). Infants with early first-degree heart block noted on fetal ultrasound should be carefully monitored for progression with collaboration between the obstetrician and pediatric cardiology team. A fetal echocardiogram should be performed for any evidence for congenital heart disease as heart block may be the first indication. Studies have been performed at the utilization of various medications and treatments (e.g., maternal steroids, immunoglobin) to the mother to help minimize the risk of progression of heart block with mostly inconclusive results. Once the fetus progresses to third-degree or complete heart block, the fetal heart rate may be too low for hemodynamic stability and may result in the development of hydrops fetalis. Early work has been performed in the creation of fetal pacing that may provide promise to prevent the development of hydrops fetalis and provide a bridge to a term delivery; however, this technology is not clinically available at this time. If possible, it is recommended to keep the fetus in utero for as long as possible with close monitoring for any worsening developments or hydropic features. During this time, planning should occur among the team to determine delivery options and the need for immediate pacing via a temporary wire. Eventually, the infant will need a permanent pacing system.

For fetal tachyarrhythmias, similar methodologies of diagnosis are needed using M-mode echocardiography, Doppler, or rarely, fetal magnetocardiography. In most instances, M-mode provides a very clear picture of atrial and ventricular contractions and can even provide indication of premature beats. Premature atrial contractions are commonly seen in the fetus and can sometimes lead to tachyarrhythmias such as an atrial tachycardia or atrial flutter with a rhythmic 2:1 or 3:1 conduction to the ventricle (see Fig. 20.1). This results in varying ectopic beats followed by a rapid, sustained rhythm much like the scenario presented. The fetus may also have a reentrant form of supraventricular tachycardia. Frequently recurrent or persistent episodes of tachycardia may begin to have detrimental effects on the fetus and could lead to hydrops fetalis. In such situations, the treatment team must initiate medical management via the mother.

Therefore, the treatment of the fetus involves the management of two patients, the mother and the fetus. The generally accepted first-line treatment for fetal tachyarrhythmias is the use of digoxin at relatively high doses in the mother to achieve appropriate levels within the fetal heart. The mother should be monitored for signs of digoxin toxicity and the fetus should be evaluated for successful management of arrhythmia. Other medications including flecainide, sotalol, and even amiodarone have been used for arrhythmia management. The side effects of these medications may be significant in the mother and all can be proarrhythmic. Mothers require careful monitoring, and in many cases, hospitalization on telemetry and daily ECG monitoring. Again, attempts at keeping the fetus in utero until term delivery are highly preferred. After the infant is delivered, medical management can be tailored if needed based on medications previously used but also have the luxury of oral availability.

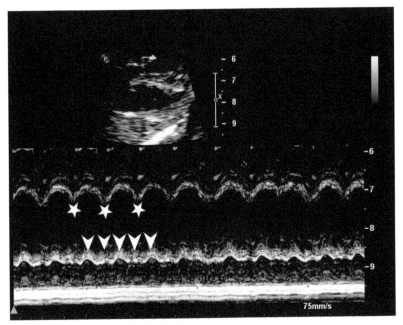

FIGURE 20.1 Fetal M-mode arrhythmia diagnosis.

Picture demonstrates an M-mode demonstration of wall movement in a fetal echocardiogram over time. The contraction of the ventricular wall is depicted on the top line (stars). The contraction of the atrial wall is depicted in the middle line (arrowheads). There are more atrial contractions at a rapid pace than ventricular contractions suggesting an atrial arrhythmia.

Given the importance of managing both mother and fetus during fetal arrhythmia, a clear communication plan and strategy should be set forth for the team and for the patient. Working through the various decision points and keeping everyone informed and updated to changes helps. This often involves different groups of individuals in different parts of the medical establishment. Special care must be taken to keep the entire team "in the loop" that requires effective coordination.

Suggested reading

Batra AS, Balaji S. Fetal arrhythmias: diagnosis and management. *Indian Pacing Electrophysiol J*. 2019;19(3):104−109. https://doi.org/10.1016/j.ipej.2019.02.007.

Wacker-Gussmann A, Strasburger JF, Cuneo BF, Wakai RT. Diagnosis and treatment of fetal arrhythmia. *Am J Perinatol*. 2014;31(7):617−628. https://doi.org/10.1055/s-0034-1372430.

A 3-month old child with complete heart block after surgery for AV canal defect

21

Case

Sorry to call you this evening but you are on call for pediatric electrophysiology right? I am the ICU fellow covering the CICU tonight along with my attending. We brought back a 3 month-old infant with Down Syndrome after surgery for an AV canal defect about an hour ago. The surgeon said that the surgery was uneventful except for a moment where the patient went into complete heart block but conduction came back after a few minutes. But just in case the surgeon left us some ventricular pacing wires. The patient has been hemodynamically stable since getting here but now we are noting that the heart rate is dropping to about 80 bpm and blood pressure is a bit low. The rhythm is steady but I'm not sure that every p wave is being conducted. I've decided to ventricular pace at 100 bpm and that has helped the blood pressure. My attending asked me to give you a call.

What am I thinking?

Surgical AV block is the most common form of acquired heart block in the young. This most commonly affects repairs where the conduction system is at risk of damage due to anatomic location such as ventricular septal defects or AV canal repairs. However, AV block has been seen in other surgical repairs in which the conduction system has not been manipulated (e.g., Fontan operation). While the most likely event here is heart block, it would be important to categorize it by using an electrocardiogram or rhythm strip (see Fig. 21.1). In scenarios where surgical heart block is a risk, cardiac surgeons will attach temporary pacing wires in case pacing is needed. Ideally, both atrial and ventricular pacing wires are provided to assist in a more physiologic approach to pacing but if ventricular wires are all that are provided, you work with what you have.

The first step is to pace to achieve hemodynamic stability. In the scenario described, pacing at a higher heart rate did assist in increasing the patient's blood pressure. An attempt should be made to match the intended heart rate of the patient by measuring the rate of atrial contraction. With a set of atrial and ventricular wires,

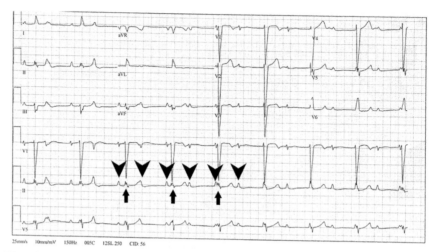

FIGURE 21.1 Surgical heart block.

ECG demonstrating third-degree or complete heart block after cardiac surgery. Sinus p waves (arrowheads) are dissociated from the QRS (arrows), which is at different rates. Widening of the QRS is likely secondary to a left bundle branch block due to surgical intervention.

it is possible to set the temporary pacemaker to an atrial sensed and ventricular paced mode that represents a more physiologic mode of pacing (see Fig. 21.2). With only ventricular wires, it is best to closely match the sinus rate with ventricular pacing alone (see Fig. 21.3). Any attempt to exceed the expected rate will eventually result in a reduced filling time of the ventricle and begin to have a negative impact on the ventricle.

Once an appropriate rate has been determined and the temporary pacemaker is set, the time clock begins, for a few reasons. First, the temporary pacing wires themselves have a short life. For this reason, pacing thresholds and sensing thresholds should be checked daily for patients requiring temporary pacing. As a point of courtesy, it is important to inform the telemetry technician (if there is one), the bedside nurse, and family members when doing so as monitors are likely to start alarming. Testing of temporary pacemakers and thresholds is best reserved for those familiar with the technology and how to troubleshoot. If thresholds begin to increase past a point of half the maximal output of the temporary pacemaker or result in unintended diaphragmatic pacing, the cardiac surgical team should be made aware about the possible need for replacement. The role of steroids or antiinflammatory agents in surgical heart block is unproven in clinical studies. Second, surgical heart block that has been demonstrated to revert to sinus rhythm within 7 days does not have a high risk of reverting back to heart block. Those that persist in heart block after 7–10 days generally require a permanent pacemaker implant as a rule of thumb.

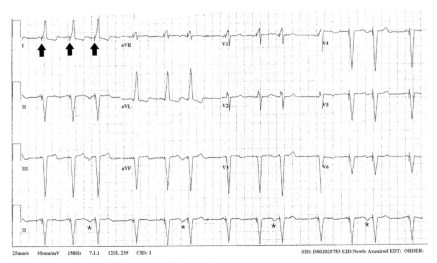

FIGURE 21.2 Atrial sensing-ventricular pacing.

ECG demonstrates a pacemaker programmed to atrial sensing with ventricular pacing. QRS
configuration is wide due to pacing activation from the right ventricular apex and artifact from
pacing signal known as a "pacing spike" (arrows) precedes the QRS. This is a synchronous
mode of pacing by sensing atrial activity and inducing ventricular pacing. Atrial activity,
including premature atrial beats (asterisks), are sensed and triggers ventricular pacing.

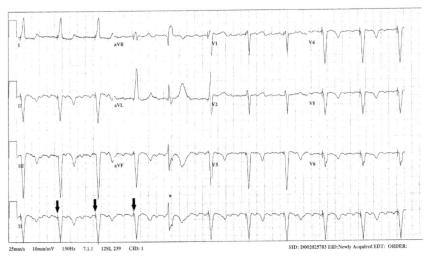

FIGURE 21.3 Asynchronous ventricular pacing.

ECG demonstrates a pacemaker programmed for ventricular pacing and sensing (i.e., VVI
mode) without sensing of atrial activity. The underlying atrial arrhythmia of atrial flutter is
ignored by the pacemaker and the ventricle is paced at a consistent set rate marked by
the pacing spike artifact (arrows). The ventricular lead is sensing as pacing is inhibited
when a premature ventricular contraction (asterisk) is sensed. Ventricular pacing
resumes after the appropriate time interval based on the set rate.

While anecdotal evidence exists of early conversion to sinus leading to late heart block and late conversion to sinus rhythm after permanent pacemaker placement, the rule of thumb generally holds true.

The decision to implant a permanent pacemaker is not singular and should be shared with the surgeon, pediatric electrophysiologist, and family but is most often driven by the needs of the patient. In infants, this requires epicardial pacing wires, and a pacemaker can be placed in the abdomen. In older congenital heart disease patients, vascular access may preclude a transvenous system. Newer technology in the form of leadless pacemakers may be helpful in this regard but have yet to be ubiquitously adopted and carry unknown long-term consequences.

A 4-month-old postoperative ventricular septal defect with junctional ectopic tachycardia

22

Case

I have a 4 month old male who underwent VSD repair earlier today. His heart rate has been climbing all afternoon and now he is running a rate of 200. His blood pressure is soft and he has stopped peeing. The QRS complexes are narrow. I think this is some kind of SVT. I tried using adenosine. It did not slow the rhythm even slightly. If anything, he sped up with it. What do I do next?

What am I thinking?

There are three big clues from what I have heard so far, which suggests that this is not a typical reentry SVT (either atrioventricular reentry tachycardia or AV nodal reentry tachycardia).

The first is the statement that the heart rate has been "climbing" all afternoon. Reentry usually starts and stops abruptly. A gradually climbing suggests that this is not a reentry tachycardia, and is more suggestive of an automatic, focal mechanism. Abnormal automaticity is a phenomenon whereby cells other than the sinus node develop properties similar to a sinus node and can generate action potentials spontaneously. Sometimes such cells fire off beats at a rate much faster than the sinus node, thereby causing a tachycardia.

The second clue is the fact that this "SVT" did not respond to adenosine. Reentry SVT (AVRT and AVNRT) typically are terminated by blocking the AV node with adenosine. An atrial tachycardia or atrial flutter is in the differential for a narrow QRS tachycardia. However, blocking the AV node leads to transient slowing of the ventricular rate that is typically transient, and once the adenosine wears off, the ventricular rate goes back to where it used to be.

Arrhythmias in Children. https://doi.org/10.1016/B978-0-323-77907-4.00022-6

The third clue is that the QRS complex is "narrow." A postoperative arrhythmia can be either an SVT or a VT. VT would have a broad QRS complex. A narrow QRS implies this is an SVT or a high septal VT that engages into the His bundle immediately, thereby leading to a narrow QRS. The most common arrhythmia that fits this description is JET or junctional ectopic tachycardia (also known as His bundle tachycardia in Britain and Europe).

JET is most commonly seen in infants soon after major open-heart surgery in the region of the AV node. Most authorities classify JET as an SVT, although it often has features similar to VT in that AV dissociation can be present (AV association can occur in some patients, with the P wave just after the QRS complex).

I would ask the caller to send me a copy of the 12 lead or monitor strip of the rhythm. Careful examination often reveals the dissociated P waves (see Fig. 22.1). In some patients, P waves can be hard to see. In such cases, it may be possible to do an ECG incorporating the atrial electrogram. Many postoperative patients come back from the OR with temporary atrial and ventricular pacing wires. Attaching one of the leads of the ECG to the atrial wire can give an atrial electrogram deflection on the ECG (see Figure 4.3).

Having made the diagnosis, I would then focus on management. Management is based on three main factors. Firstly, postoperative JET is usually self-limited, and goes away after 2–3 days. Secondly, JET can severely impact the cardiac output

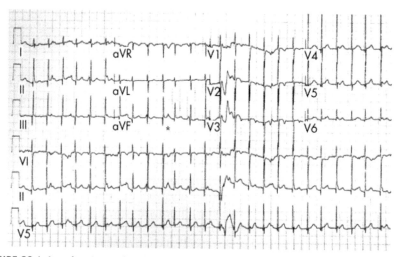

FIGURE 22.1 Junctional ectopic tachycardia.

ECG demonstrates a junctional tachycardia with atrial dissociation. As the atrial rhythm and junctional rhythm are dissociated from each other, there are occasions where the sinus P wave is able to capture the junction (asterisk) bringing the next QRS closer to the previous QRS than the standard junctional rate. This dissociation combined with tachycardia can lead to hemodynamic compromise.

and lead to major hemodynamic compromise. Thirdly, although it arises from the region of the AV node, AV conduction is usually preserved in patients with JET.

Since JET is an automatic focal arrhythmia, there is no point in trying to stop it with maneuvers like overdrive pacing or even electrical cardioversion. In fact, cardioversion may worsen things as it "weakens" the cardiac muscle, without any antiarrhythmic benefit, and therefore, is important to avoid.

As JET is an abnormal automatic focus, it is important to reduce all catecholaminergic stimulation. Such medications typically increase the rate due to their positive chronotropic effects. A careful inventory of all vasoactive medications with weaning of such medication is useful. Sometimes this is easier said than done as infants who have recently undergone a major heart surgery may have poor ventricular contractility and a certain amount of inotropic support may be critical. In such cases, one has to try and strike a balance without being overaggressive in weaning these inotropes. The same principle also applies to all vasodilators (milrinone, nitroprusside, etc.) since any lowering of the BP leads to the production of endogenous catecholamines.

Temperature can be a major driver of the heart rate and attempts to reduce the child's temperature can be very important. In fact, most babies who develop JET come from the OR in a slower junctional rhythm. During surgery, their temperature is usually kept low and hypothermic. It is the gradual rise in temperature and the tendency to overshoot and become febrile that seems to be the main driver of the tachycardia in many infants. Therefore, reducing the body temperature can be a vital part of the management. This can be accomplished in a multitude of ways: cool cloths laid on the patient, stripping the patient, lowering the room temperature, placing the baby on a cooling blanket, etc. temperatures as low as 32°C have been described, although the lower temperatures can cause a shivering reflex that generates heat and negates the cooling. This must be managed to be overcome if needed by using paralytic agents). All this presupposes that the child will remain on a ventilator for the duration of the arrhythmia.

Antiarrhythmic agents have a significant role to play. The goal of antiarrhythmic therapy, similar to cooling, is to slow the rate of tachycardia. The two main drugs that have been used in the context of JET are IV procainamide and IV amiodarone (with less frequent reports of IV esmolol). There have been no studies comparing the efficacy and safety of these drugs, and their use seems to be mainly driven by a physician and institutional preference. Most institutions seem to use amiodarone. However, the one study that compared the two showed that procainamide may be superior in some respects. Both medications have their drawbacks, with liver dysfunction being the most important one for amiodarone and potential for seizures in those who receive an overdose of IV procainamide. Both drugs are given as an initial bolus followed by an infusion, which is titrated to achieve the appropriate rate.

It is important to keep in mind that neither amiodarone nor procainamide appears to fundamentally change the rhythm. They are mainly used as rate control drugs while the spontaneous resolution of the JET is awaited. A new drug that shows promise to actually impact the abnormal automaticity and "convert" the rhythm to sinus is ivabradine. However, experience with its use in children is limited; moreover, it is not available for IV use. As most patients are unable to be fed or take medications through the gastric route immediately after cardiac surgery, this severely limits the usefulness of this novel drug.

Lastly, once the rate has been reduced with the above measures, one should be able to institute atrial pacing at a rate slightly above the rate of the native rhythm. The advantage of this is to provide AV synchrony, with a significant improvement in blood pressure and cardiac output (see Fig. 22.2). Daily or twice daily cessation of pacing to see if the native rhythm has converted to sinus is recommended. This usually takes about 2−3 days. There is often a period of alternate sinus and junctional rhythm with a gradual reduction in the periods of junctional rhythm and an increase in the periods of sinus rhythm before the arrhythmia completely resolves. The junctional rhythm itself does not pose an issue as long as there is no hemodynamic compromise (see Figure 1.4). After getting control of the rhythm and improving the cardiac output using the methods described earlier, the rest of the management becomes a waiting game.

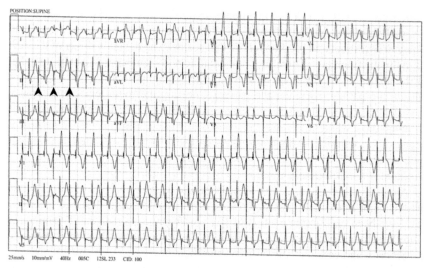

FIGURE 22.2 Overdrive atrial pacing for postoperative junctional ectopic tachycardia.

ECG demonstrating atrial pacing at approximately 150 bpm in a patient with a history of tetralogy of Fallot postoperative with underlying right bundle branch block. Atrial pacing spike is noted just before P wave (arrowheads). Atrial pacing must exceed the rate of the junctional ectopic tachycardia to maintain AV synchrony. Other measures to slow the junctional ectopic rate are often required.

A 10-year old child with a pacemaker who is dizzy and had a syncope episode

Case

Good evening, I am calling from the emergency room with a 10-year old girl with congenital heart disease that is followed at another center outside the state who has a pacemaker and had a syncopal episode. She is on vacation with her family visiting one of the local national parks and she passed out while they were on a short hike. Her mother states that she wasn't feeling well this morning and was complaining of feeling tired, but they thought maybe it was just jet lag from the flight over. After she passed out on the hike, it appears that every few minutes or so she gets really dizzy and lightheaded and then comes back to normal. Her mother says that last time the pacemaker was checked was about 18 months ago, they had missed some of the appointments. At her last appointment, the cardiologist said that they were seeing a change in one of the leads but that it was "stable for now." I can't get a hold of her primary cardiologist. Her heart rate seems fine but irregular. I got a chest X-ray and I see a lot of wires and clips from her surgery but I don't see a pacemaker in her chest. I'm wondering if you can somehow check the device to make sure it's working?

What am I thinking?

When I hear about a patient with a pacemaker who is having syncopal episodes, the first thing I need to know is if the device is functioning as intended. For patients that are known to our service, there may be clues from the previous visits such as a changing lead impedance (the resistance to the flow of current through the pacing lead. If too high, this may indicate a break or fracture in the lead (see Fig. 28.2). If too low, it may indicate a break in the insulation around the lead) or changes in sensing (sensing is the ability of the pacemaker to recognize or "sense" the patient's own native beats) or pacing thresholds (threshold is the lowest amount of current put out by the pacemaker that can reliably electrically activate the chamber in which it is

Arrhythmias in Children. https://doi.org/10.1016/B978-0-323-77907-4.00023-8

placed). These are all things we check when patients come in for their pacemaker follow-up visits. In the case of a patient unknown to us, the most important thing is to establish what type of device (and which company manufactured it) the patient has implanted to determine the appropriate device programmer to use to interrogate the device. Pacemaker patients are given a card that they should carry with them as an identification card with the information about the device and leads, including the implantation date. In case a family is unaware of the type of device, a radiopaque identification marker can be identified on radiograph and can help. Otherwise, trial and error with various pacemaker programmers can allow for the determination of the right programmer to use.

It is important to know that sometimes, the pacemaker is not in the chest. This is often the case for younger pediatric patients who have pacemakers implanted in the abdomen. In such patients, the leads are placed epicardially (touching the outer epicardial heart surface) as opposed to the traditional adult placement with a generator in the upper left chest and transvenous leads.

Pacemakers have two main functions—to sense and to pace. Previously, I mentioned the concept of the pacemaker "functioning as intended" which was a specific choice of words. It is rare for a pacemaker to not function due to a defect in design or manufacturing. However, pacemakers may function with normal system behavior without getting the intended result. An example would be a concept of oversensing where the device interprets a waveform (e.g., T wave) as a ventricular contraction and decides not to pace the heart. This can happen if the number setting the sensitivity level of the device is too low (a low number indicates the pacemaker can "sense" even smaller potentials, i.e., it is oversensitive). Another mechanism, and more likely scenario, is a failing lead that does not allow the output of the pacemaker to capture the heart.

Pacemaker leads will fail over time, hence the need for routine follow-up. Indicators of a failing lead may be a rising impedance value (too high would indicate a severe resistance to current flow as happens if the lead is fracture) and changes in pacing threshold (higher than expected current needed to activate the heart chamber, which implies there is a problem a the point of contact between the lead and the heart). Radiographs can be helpful in epicardial leads to help identify areas of lead fracture. Comparisons to previously obtained radiographs can be helpful to identify changes. Lead fractures can cause intermittent loss of capture due to intermittent connection through the fractured lead. This can happen with changes in position or movement, particularly with abdominal implants and epicardial leads. In some patients, pacing may be intermittent and the patient may have episodes of dizziness that may be the manifestation of intermittent loss of pacing.

Actions will depend on the interrogation of the device that is performed by the pediatric cardiology or electrophysiology service, often in conjunction with a device representative from the company. Most hospitals are equipped with device interrogation systems that will allow for evaluation and reprogramming of the device as needed. In the meantime, clinical support of the patient is the first step. If there is a concern of inadequate heart rate or bradycardia resulting in hemodynamic instability, providing medications such as a chronotropic agent can assist with keeping the intrinsic heart rate up while the pacemaker is being evaluated. In some cases, programming changes on the device can result in more consistent capture and a steady heart rate. If the issue is related to an oversensing issue, this can be overcome by making the pacemaker less sensitive (make the sensing number larger) or by completely removing the pacemaker's ability to sense, that is, a pacing only set up. Another way to disable the sensing function in most pacemakers is by placing a device-specific, high-powered magnet over the device that places it into a "magnet mode" and results in a pacing mode with no ability to sense. This mode results in the pacing of the heart (usually the ventricle) with no sensing. On some occasions, the lead will require to be changed out and a new lead placed. In such scenarios, the patient should be supported and observed until a corrective procedure can take place.

Suggested reading

Epstein AE, DiMarco JP, Ellenbogen KA, et al. ACC/AHA/HRS 2008 guidelines for device-based therapy of cardiac rhythm abnormalities: a report of the American College of Cardiology/American Heart Association Task Force on Practice Guidelines (writing committee to revise the ACC/AHA/NASPE 2002 guideline update for implantation of cardiac pacemakers and Antiarrhythmia devices) developed in collaboration with the American Association for Thoracic Surgery and Society of Thoracic Surgeons [published correction appears in J Am Coll Cardiol. 2009 Apr 21;53(16):1473] [published correction appears in J Am Coll Cardiol. 2009 Jan 6;53(1):147] *J Am Coll Cardiol.* 2008;51(21):e1−e62. https://doi.org/10.1016/j.jacc.2008.02.032.

Epstein AE, DiMarco JP, Ellenbogen KA, et al. 2012 ACCF/AHA/HRS focused update incorporated into the ACCF/AHA/HRS 2008 guidelines for device-based therapy of cardiac rhythm abnormalities: a report of the American College of Cardiology Foundation/American Heart Association Task Force on Practice Guidelines and the Heart Rhythm Society. *J Am Coll Cardiol.* 2013;61(3):e6−e75. https://doi.org/10.1016/j.jacc.2012.11.007.

An 11-year-old child resuscitated from sudden collapse, found to have a long QT on ECG

Case

Hi, I'm calling from the ER. We have an 11-year old who "collapsed" while at the park with his family. The family called 911, started CPR, but by the time the ambulance came he improved, and they did not have to do CPR or shock him. He looks OK now but his ECG computer read says his QT is prolonged. Please help.

What am I thinking?

A computer read that says prolonged QT is a cause for concern, but the computer can make glaring mistakes sometimes. A diagnosis of long QT syndrome is a life-changing one and has to be made with care and consideration. The computer read has to be confirmed by manual measurement. That said, in this specific case, the index of suspicion that this is a true case of long QT is high because of the presentation with collapse.

Long QT syndrome is an inherited channelopathy (a disorder of the cardiac ion channels) making the patient vulnerable to episodes of an unusual form of ventricular tachycardia called Torsades des pointes (TdP) (see Fig. 24.1). TdP can cause death, and a shock can successfully restore sinus rhythm. However, patients can have nonsustained self-terminated episodes of TdP and therefore may spontaneously recover from a "collapse" without a shock. Another confounding presentation is the likelihood of presenting with a "seizure." A TdP episode causes brain anoxia and, as a result, the patient has an anoxic seizure. When the TdP ceases, the blood supply to the brain resumes, the seizure stops, and the patient wakes up. In such an instance, it is easy to overlook the heart and go full tilt investigating the neurologic system.

A big confounder in teens and preteens is vasovagal syncope that is so much more common in this age group. Vasovagal syncope is a fainting episode with transient loss of consciousness due to transient low blood pressure. Studies have shown that 99% of

Arrhythmias in Children. https://doi.org/10.1016/B978-0-323-77907-4.00024-X

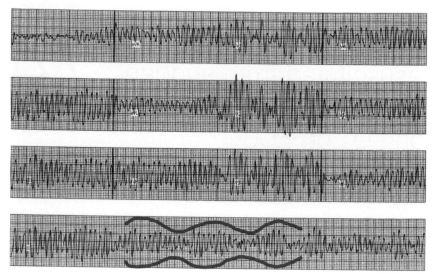

FIGURE 24.1 Torsades de pointes.

ECG demonstrating Torsades de pointes. Torsades is classically described as a twisting of ventricular arrhythmia around a point much like a party ribbon configuration (red lines).

faints in teens and preteens are due to vasovagal syncope (see Chapter 16). So, on the one hand, we have a rare life-threatening disorder (long QT) and, on the other hand, we have a benign condition that is common and almost never causes life-threatening consequences. Making a mistake either way could have terrible consequences for this child. Disregarding long QT put his life in danger, but mistakenly diagnosing long QT gives him a bad medical label to carry that can be hard to remove.

The history of the event that happened can be one of the most important aspects. If the "collapse" happened while he was running or actively playing and excited, the bias tilts toward a lethal condition like long QT and away from vasovagal syncope. A family history of someone else in the immediate family who died in a "sudden" or "unexplained" or "inadequately explained" manner further increases the index of suspicion. Family history of a "seizure-disorder" is also suspicious due to the factors discussed above.

TdP in long QT is often brought about during exercise or during a sudden alarming event, especially sudden noise such as a wakeup alarm or a fire alarm. Long QT also has a predisposition to swimming and unexplained drownings. A specific question to ask is whether there is a family history of deafness. A rare form of long QT called the Jervell and Lange-Nielsen syndrome is associated with deafness.

The ECG obtained is a crucial piece of evidence. The QT should be measured and then corrected using a formula (Bazett's formula). A QTC >460 ms in boys and >480 ms in girls is considered abnormal. It is important to also look at the "shape" of the T waves. They can be bizarre in long QT syndrome (see Figs. 24.2–24.4).

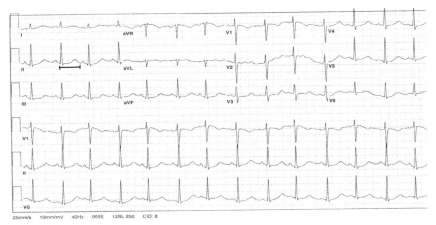

FIGURE 24.2 Long QT Syndrome, type 1 pattern.

ECG demonstrates sinus rhythm with a prolonged QT (measurement) with a broad-based T wave. This is the most common form of Long QT Syndrome and is secondary to a potassium channel mutation.

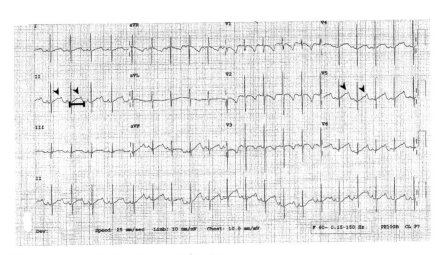

FIGURE 24.3 Long QT Syndrome, type 2 pattern.

ECG demonstrates sinus rhythm with a prolonged QT (measurement) with a notched T wave (arrowheads). This is the second most common form of Long QT Syndrome and is secondary to a potassium channel mutation.

Another important factor to consider is that extraneous factors like electrolyte imbalance and certain medications can lead to prolongation of the QT interval. Common offenders are hypokalemia, hypocalcemia, and hypomagnesemia. A long list of drugs (available at www.crediblemeds.org) can lead to QT prolongation. Certain

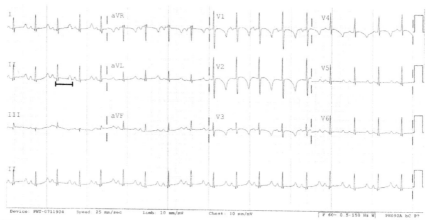

FIGURE 24.4 Long QT Syndrome, type 3 pattern.

ECG demonstrates sinus rhythm with a prolonged QT (measurement) with a long isoelectric segment and late peaking T wave. This is secondary to a sodium channel mutation.

brain conditions like migraines, resuscitative hypothermia, and intracranial hemorrhage can cause QT prolongation. Lastly, the QT can be prolonged after any resuscitation with its profound fluid shifts and potential cardiac trauma. If none of these common confounders are present and the QT is still prolonged, the possibility of congenital long QT syndrome is high. To confound matters further, the QT interval may not always be prolonged in patients with congenital long QT syndrome!

Given the above factors, I would have a low threshold for admitting this child for observation unless there was overwhelming evidence to the contrary suggesting this "collapse" was not a true "collapse" and merely a vasovagal faint.

Suggested reading

Ackerman MJ. Genotype-phenotype relationships in congenital long QT syndrome. *J Electrocardiol.* 2005;38(4 Suppl):64–68. https://doi.org/10.1016/j.jelectrocard. 2005.06.018.

Crediblemeds.org. *Crediblemeds: Home*; 2020. Available at: https://crediblemeds.org/. Accessed November 16, 2020.

A 12-year old with hypertrophic cardiomyopathy presents to the emergency room with syncope

25

Case

Hi, I'm calling from the ER. We have a 12 year old boy who sees cardiology for hypertrophic cardiomyopathy (HCM). He fainted today at school during recess. He looks OK now and all vitals are stable. Do I need to do anything else or can I discharge him with a plan to be seen back by cardiology?

What am I thinking?

I am very worried about this patient. This patient needs to be admitted for further workup and observation. He has an underlying condition with a risk for lethal arrhythmias and sudden death and now he presents with fainting. Although vasovagal syncope (simple fainting) is common in kids, any fainting in a child with an underlying heart disease should be taken very seriously. In fact, in teenagers and young adults, HCM is the commonest cause of sudden death. In any patient with an underlying heart problem who presents with fainting, vasovagal syncope should only be considered after every effort has been taken to make sure the patient could not have had a lethal arrhythmia that aborted. In fact, just as arrhythmias can begin suddenly for inexplicable reasons, they can also stop suddenly and inexplicably.

Since this patient has already been seeing a cardiologist and has a diagnosis of HCM, presumably we already have some history. It would be important to review the previous notes of this child. It would also be important to ask the family if the child has been sick recently or had an intercurrent illness. HCM is characterized by abnormal thickening of the ventricles, which, in turn, makes them less compliant (stiff), and thereby can limit their cardiac output. An intercurrent illness associated with diarrhea, vomiting, or poor oral intake and associated dehydration can be very poorly tolerated by such patients. The fact that the child went to school suggests there was no intercurrent illness, but it would be important to be sure.

It is also important to try to tease out what the child was doing when he passed out. Was he running in the playground or playing with friends? Syncope associated with physical exertion generally suggests a lethal arrhythmia, while syncope at rest or standing still is less suggestive. It is also important to ask whether any onlookers who observed the fainting noted seizure-like activity or whether there was incontinence of the bladder/bowels. The presence of any of these features would be highly concerning for a serious arrhythmia in this patient.

A thorough, cardiovascular-focused, examination in patients with HCM includes listening carefully for any murmurs. Additionally, it is important to listen with the patient standing, squatting, and while standing after having been squatting. The last maneuver can help "unmask" a dynamic left ventricular outflow tract obstruction, if present.

If the child was on a cardiac monitor while being observed in the ER, it is important to see if he has been having any premature ventricular complexes (PVCs) or even small runs of any arrhythmia. If not already done, the most critical tests to order are an ECG (see Fig. 25.1) and an echocardiogram. However, even if they are unchanged from previous studies, it is important to not be falsely reassured.

A cardiac MRI (CMR) should be considered. CMR has been shown to be more sensitive to unusual forms of hypertrophy and localized forms of hypertrophy. In

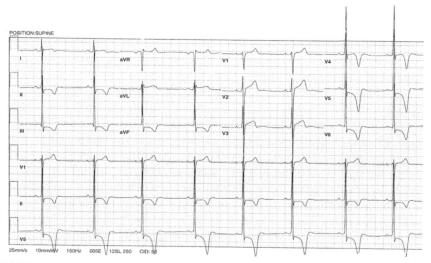

FIGURE 25.1 ECG findings in hypertrophic cardiomyopathy.

ECG demonstrates sinus rhythm with tall R waves in the lateral precordial leads (V4–V6) suggestive of left ventricular hypertrophy coupled with ST-segment depression and T-wave inversion in the inferior (II, III, aVF) and lateral precordial leads. These findings are highly suggestive of hypertrophic cardiomyopathy.

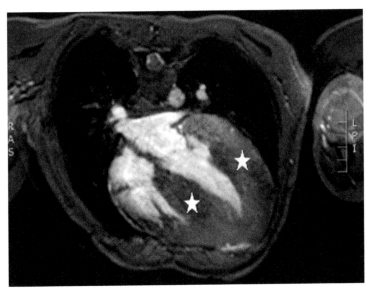

FIGURE 25.2 Cardiac MRI of hypertrophic cardiomyopathy.

Image taken from the cardiac MRI of a patient with hypertrophic cardiomyopathy clearly demonstrating the extremely thickened walls of the ventricle (stars). The abnormal thickness can impede blood flow as well as contain scar tissue, both of which can result in sudden cardiac arrest.

addition, a late gadolinium-enhanced MRI can reveal scars in the myocardium, and the extent and severity of such scars has been shown to correlate with electrical vulnerability with lethal arrhythmias (see Fig. 25.2).

An exercise test should be considered as arrhythmias may be "induced" by exercise, and that would point to the need for aggressive treatment. While the electrocardiogram can be difficult to interpret at times, a tracing of the rhythm can provide the diagnosis or provide clues to appropriately identify the arrhythmia.

Consultation with a pediatric electrophysiologist is strongly advised. The main purpose is to decide this child's risk for sudden death due to a lethal ventricular arrhythmia. If this risk is thought to be high (generally taken as a likelihood for lethal arrhythmias of >6% over 5 years), this child will need an implantable defibrillator to be placed to protect him in the instance of repeated ventricular arrhythmia.

Suggested reading

Balaji S, DiLorenzo MP, Fish FA, et al. Risk factors for lethal arrhythmic events in children and adolescents with hypertrophic cardiomyopathy and an implantable defibrillator: an international multicenter study. *Heart Rhythm*. 2019;16(10):1462–1467. https://doi.org/10.1016/j.hrthm.2019.04.040.

A 13-year old with repaired tetralogy of Fallot with frequent PVCs

26

Case

I have a 13 year old in my office who is here for a routine well child evaluation. She has had cardiac surgery to repair a tetralogy of Fallot when she was under a year of age. When I examined her, I could hear an irregular rhythm. So, we did an ECG and it shows two premature ventricular contractions (PVCs). I'd like her to come see you. How soon should she see you and are there any other tests or treatment she should have in the meantime? Also, she is a swimmer and has a swim competition this weekend. Can she be allowed to swim?

What am I thinking?

Tetralogy of Fallot is one of the most common cyanotic congenital heart diseases and is usually diagnosed in infancy. The key defects in the heart are a large ventricular septal defect and pulmonary stenosis. The pulmonary stenosis can be at multiple levels (valve, below the valve or above the valve, or a combination of these). Almost all children undergo corrective surgery that consists of closing the VSD and relief of the pulmonary stenosis. In the process of relieving the obstruction out of the right ventricle, the competency of the pulmonary valve can be affected resulting in significant pulmonary valve regurgitation, which leads to enlargement and stretching of the right ventricle. On the other hand, the pulmonary stenosis may be inadequately relieved leaving the patient with significant obstruction out of the right ventricle. Both these issues (pulmonary stenosis and or regurgitation) place stress on the right ventricle. The development of significant ventricular arrhythmias is an important long-term consequence of this right ventricular stress. In extreme cases, the patient may develop ventricular tachycardia or fibrillation leading to collapse and even sudden death. When a primary care physician tells me this child with tetralogy of Fallot repair has PVCs, I must decide: are these ectopic beats a benign and unrelated finding or is this child at significant risk of going into ventricular arrhythmias that could be potentially life-threatening?

Arrhythmias in Children. https://doi.org/10.1016/B978-0-323-77907-4.00026-3

Questions I would ask the pediatrician are: how is the child doing? Has she experienced any symptoms like syncope (especially during physical exercise), difficulty breathing or chest pain with exercise, or random episodes of the feeling that her heart is racing? A negative answer to these questions would be highly reassuring. A positive answer, especially to the fainting question, may prove highly concerning with the need for the child to be seen right away.

I would also ask for the ECG right away for review. I would pay particular attention to the rhythm and the QRS complexes as a longer QRS duration has been found to be associated with poor outcomes. I would also look at the PVCs to see if they are monomorphic (same appearance), which is more common, or multiform (differing appearance) potentially implying that the ectopic beats are arising from more than one spot and is more concerning for a diffuse disease process (see Figs. 26.1 and 26.2).

The question of when to see her will depend on the above questions. If she is symptomatic especially with fainting, light-headedness, or chest pain during exercise, I would see her immediately. If the answers are reassuring, there is no urgency and other tests may be pursued before she is seen in the clinic. The most important tests would be an echocardiogram and an ECG monitor of some kind like the Holter or any of the newer styles of ECG monitors (see Chapter 5). The more abnormal these tests are, the more concerned I would be for progressing disease. If she gives

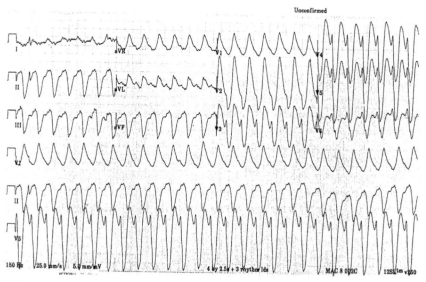

FIGURE 26.1 Monomorphic ventricular tachycardia in tetralogy of fallot patient.

ECG demonstrates a monomorphic (single morphology QRS) wide complex tachycardia in a patient with tetralogy of Fallot. Although symptomatic, the patient was able to tolerate the tachycardia without hemodynamic compromise.

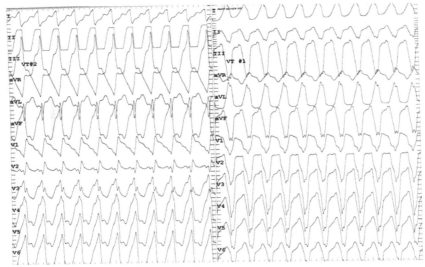

FIGURE 26.2 Multiple forms of ventricular tachycardia in tetralogy of fallot patient.

ECG demonstrates two separate forms of ventricular tachycardia in a patient with tetralogy of Fallot while performing an electrophysiology study. Note the different morphologies among the two ventricular arrhythmias. Both tachycardias resulted in a significant hemodynamic compromise to the patient.

a history of symptoms during exercise, I would also strongly consider doing an exercise test to see if it induces a significant arrhythmia.

Sports participation can be a tricky question. There is no need to unnecessarily alarm the pediatrician, the child, or her parents. However, I want to make sure she is not being placed at any unnecessary risk. The answer to sports participation will depend on the answers the pediatrician gives to my questions above. If her symptoms are concerning (syncope, lightheadedness, or chest pain, especially with exercise), I would request that she avoid sports like swimming until she has been evaluated by a cardiologist. If she is doing fine otherwise and these PVCs were an incidental detection, I would be fine with her continuing to swim and do other sports while the evaluation proceeds. Having said this, it would be prudent to make sure there is an AED present on the premises where she exercises, as a back-up safety measure (see Chapter 27).

Suggested reading

Atallah J, Gonzalez Corcia MC, Walsh EP. Participating members of the pediatric and congenital electrophysiology society. Ventricular arrhythmia and life-threatening events in patients with repaired tetralogy of Fallot [published correction appears in Am J Cardiol. 2020 Nov 6] *Am J Cardiol.* 2020;132:126−132. https://doi.org/10.1016/j.amjcard.2020.07.012.

A 15-year old presents after successful resuscitation with an AED

27

Case

Hi this is the ER attending calling. I have an ambulance on route from a local high school. They are telling me that they have a 15-year old male who was at wrestling practice and collapsed. The coaches were trained in CPR and said that the boy was not breathing and did not have a pulse, reportedly. They had an AED at the gym and hooked it up to him. The system stated that a "shock was advised" so they actually shocked the kid! The kid has a pulse but was down for about 10 minutes. The EMTs tell me that the kid feels fine and wants to go back to practice. I told them to go ahead and bring him in but I doubt this is real. He's too young to have a cardiac arrest, right?

What am I thinking?

As has been previously demonstrated, sudden cardiac arrest in a young person is a very real though rare event. My first thought is to bring this adolescent to medical attention immediately and start a workup to understand the details of the event, hopefully leading to an etiology.

When a young person suffers a cardiac arrest and is unsuccessfully resuscitated it is devastating not only for the family, but for the community. Pediatric cardiologists are often inundated with patient visits and phone consultations after such events as families are concerned that the same event could happen to their child. Their anxiety, while understandable, is not born out in the statistics as sudden cardiac death occurs in an estimated 1 per 100,000 persons when excluding infants and those above 18 years. Unfortunately, etiologies for the sudden cardiac death in the young is often undetermined.

What is encouraging, in this case, is that the coaches were appropriately trained in resuscitation and had an automated external defibrillator (AED) on the premises. A rapid and coordinated first-response can be life-saving. While we often hear of the shocking events of unexplained deaths in the young, we do not often hear about the "saves" that occur based on the actions of bystanders. Empowering yourself with

Arrhythmias in Children. https://doi.org/10.1016/B978-0-323-77907-4.00027-5

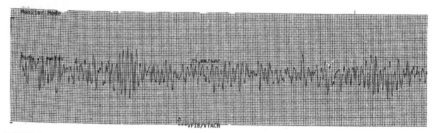

FIGURE 27.1 Automated external defibrillator tracing.

Single lead demonstration of ventricular fibrillation arrhythmia downloaded from an automated external defibrillator (AED). Certain AED devices have the capability of recording rhythm that can be critical to diagnosis.

knowledge about how to perform resuscitative measures may lead to saving someone's life. More often than not, it will be to save someone that you know or love. The American Heart Association encourages everyone to learn and administer "Hands only cardiopulmonary resuscitation (CPR)" in the event of a sudden cardiac arrest while calling for help. "Hands only CPR" can be described simply as pushing hard and fast (100 bpm) in the center of the chest and allowing for full chest recoil between every compression.

The next key to survival is becoming comfortable with an AED. Workplaces, schools, churches, nonprofits, and other public or private organizations have taken measures to incorporate AEDs for safety of their communities, but more can be done. Beyond having an AED in place, it is important for people to know when to get one and to be comfortable with how to use one. Although it may go without saying, an AED should be only used on an unconscious patient. AEDs are intended to be "user-friendly" and provide instruction as to where to apply pads and how to operate. Some will even provide instructions on how to perform CPR. With pads applied and compressions paused, an AED determines the rhythm and whether a shock would be advised (see Fig. 27.1). If a shock is advised, the user should clear the patient and press the shock button immediately followed by CPR. The AED will continue to analyze the rhythm throughout the resuscitation process and breaks from compressions should be kept to a minimum.

Investing the time to learn resuscitative measures and understanding the operation of an AED are the first steps in improving the public health of our society. Reducing the hesitancy to act in an emergency can indeed be life-saving.

Suggested reading

Atkins DL, Berger S. Improving outcomes from out-of-hospital cardiac arrest in young children and adolescents. *Pediatr Cardiol*. 2012;33(3):474−483. https://doi.org/10.1007/s00246-011-0084-8.

Kovach J, Berger S. Automated external defibrillators and secondary prevention of sudden cardiac death among children and adolescents. *Pediatr Cardiol*. 2012;33(3):402−406. https://doi.org/10.1007/s00246-012-0158-2.

Thomas VC, Shen JJ, Stanley R, Dahlke J, McPartlin S, Row L. Improving defibrillation efficiency in area schools. *Congenit Heart Dis*. 2016;11(4):359−364. https://doi.org/10.1111/chd.12375.

A 16-year-old teen with a defibrillator who received a shock

28

Case

I have a 16-year old young man with history of an aborted sudden cardiac arrest and an implanted cardioverter defibrillator (ICD) who presented to urgent care this evening. Earlier today he was playing basketball with some friends and he said that he felt someone punch him really hard in the back. He didn't know who did it so he just kept playing. Later in the evening after coming back from school he was lying on the couch watching TV. His mother called him for dinner and as he got up off the couch and started to head to the kitchen he felt a thump as though he got kicked in the chest and immediately fell to the ground. His mother saw him fall and checked to see if he was OK and he appeared fine but was in pain. She brought him in here. I have ordered a chest X-ray to check it out. Anything else I can do?

What am I thinking?

From the description of the events, it sounds like that this young man has received a "discharge" or shock from his ICD. The next question to answer is was it an "appropriate" or "inappropriate" shock? Any patient that received or is thought to have received a discharge from their ICD should have an immediate interrogation of their device (see Figs. 28.1 and 28.2). Modern ICD systems can allow for remote monitoring that allows patients to provide self-interrogation of their device that can be sent electronically to their electrophysiologist. However, such systems do not allow for programming of the device that may be required. Therefore, it is not uncommon for individuals with ICDs who have received shocks to seek care in an emergency room or urgent care.

In the event of an appropriate discharge for ICD, it is important for us to determine the etiology of the arrhythmia resulting in the treatment. For those with a known diagnosis, this may mean a breakthrough arrhythmia that was intended to be controlled by medications. I often ask questions around medication compliance or recent changes in dosage. In some patients, the ICD may have been placed as a

Arrhythmias in Children. https://doi.org/10.1016/B978-0-323-77907-4.00028-7

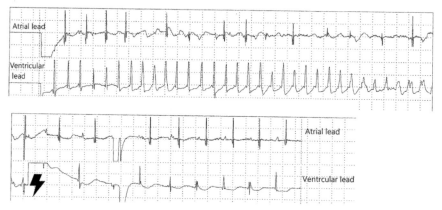

FIGURE 28.1 Implantable cardioverter defibrillator appropriate shock.

Downloaded information from an implantable cardioverter-defibrillator (ICD) of a patient who received a shock. The top strip depicts the atrial lead and the bottom strip depicts the ventricular lead. A rapid ventricular rhythm (~300 bpm) is sensed in the ventricular lead with dissociation of the atrial lead consistent with a ventricular tachycardia. The ICD detects the arrhythmia, charges, and delivers (lightning bolt) a 25 J shock to terminate the arrhythmia followed by an atrial sensed and ventricular sensed rhythm.

primary prevention for a diagnosis of concern (namely, they are known to have an underlying heart condition that puts them at risk for lethal arrhythmias and sudden death), in which case the system worked as designed. But to prevent further episodes of arrhythmia, I might consider a medication. An important decision is whether to admit for an in-hospital observation and monitoring while medication changes are being made. The most likely answer is yes, as that is often the safest course. A chest radiograph should be obtained to eliminate any potential device or lead problems (see Fig. 23.1). Interrogation of the ICD should reveal the shocks delivered as well as a recording of the preceding rhythm, its detection, and eventual rhythm post-shock. This is critical to determine the arrhythmia and possibly the initiation that can guide counseling and therapy.

In the event of an inappropriate discharge for ICD, it is critical to understand what may have resulted in the ICD misinterpreting the rhythm. Often this is the result of some interference of sensing on the lead. This can result from lead fractures, external interference, or failure of connection of the lead to the generator. ICD lead fractures can be demonstrated on chest radiograph and are a good place to start. Interrogation of the device using the appropriate interrogator is the next step. As lead fractures and lead connection issues may be intermittent, it is helpful to do chest and arm movement to coincide with a live interrogation to determine if there is any artifact noted on the lead. If there is a lead problem, it is important to deactivate the ICD. This can be done by programming through the interrogator but now we leave the patient with a nonfunctioning ICD. If the patient is known to be at risk for arrhythmia, this may require the need for external defibrillation.

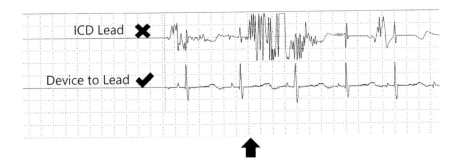

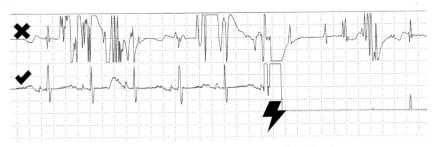

FIGURE 28.2 Implantable cardioverter defibrillator inappropriate shock.

Downloaded information from an implantable cardioverter-defibrillator (ICD) of a patient who received a shock. The top strip represents the electrical signal from the ICD lead (marked with X) and the bottom strip represents the electrical signal between the device to the lead mimicking a single-lead ECG (marked with checkmark). Noise is noted on the ICD lead that the device detects as ventricular fibrillation (detected at arrow) while the bottom strip clearly demonstrates a normal rhythm. The device charges and delivers a 10 J shock (lightning bolt) based on the misinterpretation of noise on the lead as ventricular arrhythmia. This was considered an inappropriate shock due to lead fracture.

This can be done in hospital but for home, there are less available alternatives. Sometimes we have to consider use of a wearable defibrillator if the lead cannot be attended to right away or even a home automated external defibrillator. In most cases, we try and take care of these fractured leads as soon as possible.

High power magnets can also turn off the defibrillation capability of the ICD while the magnet is placed over the device. Once the magnet is removed, the device will allow for shocks. It can be useful for patients to have these magnets if there are concerns for inappropriate shocks bearing in mind the need for immediate removal if there is concern for the need of an appropriate shock. Magnets may be used by first responders or in emergency rooms but ideally this is while the patient is on a cardiac monitor to determine if there is any change in rhythm that requires intervention.

In the clinical scenario presented, I have concerns about both appropriate or inappropriate shocks. The first shock was while the teen was playing basketball that may have been an arrhythmia but difficult to say as he does not describe any further symptoms. The second shock may have been inappropriate as he was getting off the couch that usually is not arrhythmia provoking. Sometimes movement like the one described might exacerbate noise on a lead that is fractured. I would start with a chest radiograph and ask for an interrogation of the ICD as soon as possible. The use of a magnet may be acceptable in this scenario as long as the patient's rhythm is being monitored in an emergency room or intensive care type of setting. The most important next step, however, is to get the interrogation of the ICD done as expeditiously as possible. Based on our findings from the interrogation, we can make a plan of action.

Suggested reading

DeMaso DR, Neto LB, Hirshberg J. Psychological and quality-of-life issues in the young patient with an implantable cardioverter-defibrillator. *Heart Rhythm.* 2009;6(1):130−132. https://doi.org/10.1016/j.hrthm.2008.07.022.

Silka MJ, Kron J, Dunnigan A, Dick 2nd M. Sudden cardiac death and the use of implantable cardioverter-defibrillators in pediatric patients. The Pediatric Electrophysiology Society. *Circulation.* 1993;87(3):800−807. https://doi.org/10.1161/01.cir.87.3.800.

Epstein AE, DiMarco JP, Ellenbogen KA, et al. ACC/AHA/HRS 2008 guidelines for device-based therapy of cardiac rhythm abnormalities: a report of the American College of Cardiology/American Heart Association Task Force on Practice Guidelines (writing committee to revise the ACC/AHA/NASPE 2002 guideline update for implantation of cardiac Pacemakers and antiarrhythmia devices) developed in collaboration with the American Association for Thoracic Surgery and Society of Thoracic Surgeons [published correction appears in J Am Coll Cardiol. 2009 Apr 21;53(16):1473] [published correction appears in J Am Coll Cardiol. 2009 Jan 6;53(1):147] *J Am Coll Cardiol.* 2008;51(21): e1−e62. https://doi.org/10.1016/j.jacc.2008.02.032.

Epstein AE, DiMarco JP, Ellenbogen KA, et al. 2012 ACCF/AHA/HRS focused update incorporated into the ACCF/AHA/HRS 2008 guidelines for device-based therapy of cardiac rhythm abnormalities: a report of the American College of Cardiology Foundation/American Heart Association Task Force on Practice Guidelines and the Heart Rhythm Society. *J Am Coll Cardiol.* 2013;61(3):e6−e75. https://doi.org/10.1016/j.jacc.2012.11.007.

A 22-year old with history of Fontan palliation presents with mildly elevated heart rate

29

Case

Hi, I'm calling you about a 22-year old female who I follow here in GI clinic due to her diagnosis of single ventricle palliation with a Fontan and her subsequent development of protein losing enteropathy. She comes in for routine follow-up and from her PLE standpoint, she's actually doing great. But today she's complaining that over the last two weeks she's been feeling very tired and has a lack of energy. I put her on a pulse oximeter in clinic and her oxygen saturation is 95%, which is what it has been in the past. But the machine is reading her heart rate at 110 bpm. I looked back on my notes and her heart rate usually runs 70–80 bpm so this seems a little fast to me. She doesn't appear dehydrated and she isn't febrile. I'm sending her for some baseline GI labs. She's been waiting for about an hour and a half due to a back up in the lab and I've kept the pulse oximeter on her finger to monitor her heart rate. It has stayed persistently at 110 bpm without any variation. I'm a little worried something might be going on.

What am I thinking?

Patients with congenital heart disease who have undergone surgical intervention are at risk for the development of arrhythmias. This is related to the development of areas of scar in areas of suture or patches that can serve as substrates for arrhythmia circuits. Arrhythmias may be atrial or ventricular in origin depending on the region of surgical work performed. For patients who have manipulation of atrial tissue such as an atrial switch procedure (Mustard or Senning) for transposition of the great arteries or the Fontan operation for single ventricle physiology, can be a set up for atrial reentrant rhythms. Patients who have had work performed in the ventricle such as tetralogy of Fallot would be at risk of ventricular tachycardia. These patients should be under the care of a pediatric or adult congenital cardiologist and/or electrophysiologist.

Arrhythmias in Children. https://doi.org/10.1016/B978-0-323-77907-4.00029-9

In the scenario presented, the patient presents with a heart rate of 110 bpm. While this rate is not exceedingly high, it is suggestive of an arrhythmia, particularly in the congenital heart patient who has undergone palliation. Persistent arrhythmias at these moderately tachycardic rates in patients with palliated heart disease may result in cardiac dysfunction. Patients can present with symptoms of congestive heart failure including fatigue, pulmonary edema, and respiratory insufficiency.

For those patients with atrial arrhythmias, the ventricular rate is dependent on the conduction through the AV node and can be protective from further symptomatology or sudden decompensation. Therefore, an atrial rate between 220 and 300 bpm that is blocked 2:1 may result in a pulse rate of 110–150 bpm. Careful analysis of the electrocardiogram can demonstrate additional P waves suggestive of an intraatrial reentrant tachycardia (IART) (see Fig. 29.1). Additional clues that an IART may be occurring is the lack of heart rate variability when in the arrhythmia (see Fig. 29.2). The consistency in the rhythm is based on the defined circuit, usually circling a valve or area of the scar. If there are changes in heart rate, they may be resulting from varying AV conduction and are usually seen as changes from 2:1 to 3:1 conduction. In some situations, AV conduction can be enhanced leading to a sudden change in rate to 1:1 conduction and hemodynamic collapse, particularly in the patient with less than normal cardiac function.

Management of the patient primarily lies in alleviating the inciting arrhythmia safely, without risk of sequelae. Patients with previously operated hearts and in an atrial arrhythmia are at the risk of thrombus formation, particularly those who have been in those arrhythmias for extended or unknown periods of time. Subsequently, it is generally recommended that those patients who have been in their arrhythmia for >48 h undergo an evaluation by imaging for thrombus, usually by transesophageal echocardiogram, before cardioversion. This is adapted from the management of atrial fibrillation. Anticoagulation and obligatory rate control for at least 2–3 weeks before cardioversion without the need of imaging could also

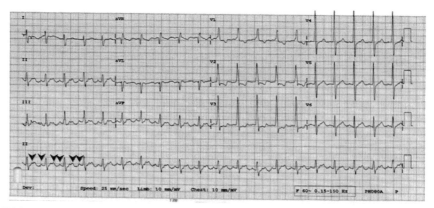

FIGURE 29.1 Intraatrial reentrant tachycardia (IART).

ECG demonstrates a mild tachycardia (~150 bpm) with a 2:1 atrial conduction. P waves are noted but with additional p waves buried within the T wave (arrowheads). Patient has a history of congenital heart disease s/p surgical repair.

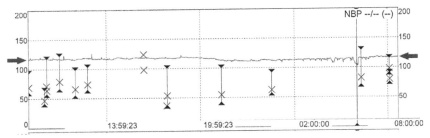

FIGURE 29.2 Persistent rate of intraatrial reentrant tachycardia (IART).

Graphical depiction of heart rate over time in a patient with AV canal status-post surgical repair and IART admitted to the hospital. Heart rate is on the Y-axis with time on the X-axis. Note the minimal change in heart rate (red arrows) at around 120 bpm over an extended time frame including during sleeping hours.

be considered though remaining in the atrial arrhythmia for a palliated congenital heart disease patient is not desirable. One possible rare exception is the patient with complete heart block and a pacemaker in whom device programming can provide rate control. The overarching goal, however, should be to focus on identifying patients early and addressing the rhythm sooner than later.

In preparation for transesophageal echocardiogram and/or cardioversion, careful consideration needs to be done when it comes to the specifics of anesthetics or sedation. This fact becomes important when considering management and the use of agents that may potentiate AV conduction and lead to 1:1 conduction of rapid atrial arrhythmias resulting in rapid decompensation in the patient. In the setting of these forms of arrhythmia, the patient should be prepped with cardioverter/defibrillator patches already in position on the patient and the device placed in "synched" mode set to the appropriate starting energy for cardioversion (i.e., 0.5−1 J/kg biphasic or 100−150 J in adult-sized patients) before sedation. Always ensure that the patches are applied in the appropriate positions for the patient keeping in mind that patients with congenital heart disease may also have dextrocardia. The physician performing the cardioversion should be present during induction in case immediate cardioversion is required.

In the patient with recurrences of these arrhythmias, consideration should be given to the options of chronic antiarrhythmic therapy (usually with strong antiarrhythmic agents like flecainide, sotalol, or dofetilide), intracardiac catheter ablation, or arrhythmia surgery. Several factors are taken into consideration, including suspected arrhythmia substrate, underlying anatomy, surgically modified anatomy, vascular access, and patient preferences. Often decisions are made by committee with the input of pediatric cardiologist, adult congenital cardiologist, cardiac surgeon, and electrophysiologist. The focus of ablation or surgery is to eliminate areas of conduction that are a part of the arrhythmia circuit by creating lines of the block (see Fig. 29.3). There is a risk that further ablation in an area could create additional sources for arrhythmia circuit. Recurrent or new arrhythmias are unfortunately common in this population and therefore continued follow-up is required with routine monitoring.

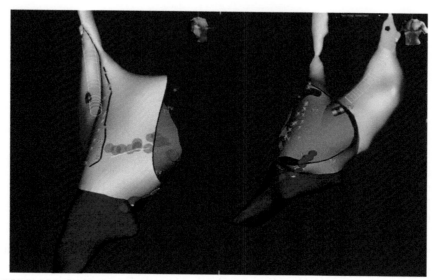

FIGURE 29.3 Electrophysiology ablation of intraatrial reentrant tachycardia.

Image is taken from an electrophysiology study and ablation in a patient with AV canal with left superior vena cava to coronary sinus status-post surgical repair using the St. Jude Ensite NavX system. Two images depict the right anterior oblique and left anterior oblique vies of the right atrium and right superior vena cava (tan), the inferior vena cava (pink), and the dilated coronary sinus (blue-green). A catheter (yellow) is depicted in the coronary sinus. A catheter (dark blue) is near the AV node. Areas marked as TV are sites on the surgically created tricuspid valve annulus. Areas marked with a green x depicts the course of the phrenic nerve. The orange and red dots are sites of ablation to create lines of the block in the circuit to eliminate reentrant atrial arrhythmias of IART.

Suggested reading

Khairy P, Van Hare GF, Balaji S, et al. PACES/HRS Expert Consensus Statement on the Recognition and Management of Arrhythmias in Adult Congenital Heart Disease: developed in partnership between the Pediatric and Congenital Electrophysiology Society (PACES) and the Heart Rhythm Society (HRS). Endorsed by the governing bodies of PACES, HRS, the American College of Cardiology (ACC), the American Heart Association (AHA), the European Heart Rhythm Association (EHRA), the Canadian Heart Rhythm Society (CHRS), and the International Society for Adult Congenital Heart Disease (ISACHD). *Heart Rhythm.* 2014;11(10):e102−e165. https://doi.org/10.1016/j.hrthm.2014.05.009.

Thomas VC, Trivedi B. Nonfluoroscopic ablation in the setting of congenital heart disease. *J Innov Card Rhythm Manag.* 2018;9(10):3359−3364. https://doi.org/10.19102/icrm.2018.091005. Published 2018 Oct 15.

Index

Printed and bound by CPI Group (UK) Ltd, Croydon, CR0 4YY

03/10/2024

01040300-0018